3/11

D1627207

Baca Grande Library
P.O. Box 36
Crestone, CO 81131

DATE DUE

GAYLORD			PRINTED IN U.S.A.

N-8

A FIRESIDE BOOK
PUBLISHED BY SIMON & SCHUSTER

The Safe Child Book

Revised and Updated

A Commonsense Approach to Protecting Children
and Teaching Children to Protect Themselves

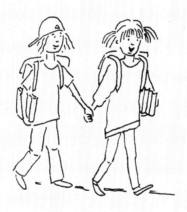

Sherryll Kraizer, Ph.D.
illustrations by Mary Kornblum

For my son, Charlie

FIRESIDE
Rockefeller Center
1230 Avenue of the Americas
New York, NY 10020

Text copyright © 1985, 1996 by Sherryll Kraizer
Illustrations copyright © 1985, 1996 by Mary Kornblum

FIRESIDE and colophon are registered trademarks
of Simon & Schuster Inc.

Designed by Gretchen Achilles

Manufactured in the United States of America

10   9   8   7   6   5   4   3   2   1

Library of Congress Cataloging-in-Publication Data
Kraizer; Sherryll Kerns.
    The safe child book: a commonsense approach to protecting
children and teaching children to protect themselves / Sherryll
Kraizer; illustrations by Mary Kornblum.
       p.   cm.
    Originally published: New York: Delacorte Press, 1985.
    Includes bibliographical references (p.   ).
    1. Child Sexual abuse—Prevention—Study and teaching—United
States.   2. Abduction—Prevention—Study and teaching—United
States.   3. Child abuse—Prevention—Study and teaching—United
States.   4. Day care centers—United States—Evaluation.   I. Title.
HQ72.U53K73   1996
362.7'6—dc20   96-20408

ISBN 0-684-81423-4

Acknowledgments

I want to thank:

My husband, Al Kraizer, for his unwavering support and encouragement of this work. He has been a friend, a critic, and a partner, always contributing energy, insight, and love.

My son, Charlie, for his humor, for challenging everything, and for teaching me what I need to know.

Barbara Binswanger, who not only saw the potential of this book but also made it possible by her support and perseverance.

Jim Charlton, my book packager, for his enthusiasm, understanding, and professionalism. Without him I would still be trying to write this book.

Sydny Miner, my editor at Simon & Schuster, for taking the work as seriously as I do.

Finally, special thanks are due all the women who have contributed their time, energy, and enthusiasm to the development of the Children Need To Know program from which this book evolved: Suzanne Adams, Margie Antal-Green, Margaret Casart, Gina Deal, Marilou Edwards, Gage Evans-Norris, Karen Farrar, Sandy Griffin, Kathy Hardison, Teresa Howes, Mady Keiley, Kathy Langston, Helen Mann, Jean Martini, Kathy Marvin, Ellen Masko, Jean Mensendick, Marilyn Miller, Valerie Norris, Betty O'Neill, Judy O'Shea, Adrian Rainey, Connie Smith, and Theresa Vigil.

Contents

Introduction

About Parents

Ambivalence is a very real part of parenting. Most parents constantly feel pulled between their guiding beliefs and principles and "reality." The decisions parents make are shaped by myriad factors, including philosophy, belief systems, history, feelings, and the opinions of others. Conflict among these creates corresponding conflict between what parents feel they should do and what they feel tempted or compelled to do. This can profoundly the affect safety of children.

For example, what parent hasn't gone through this scenario? At the end of a long afternoon of errands, having taken her two preschoolers in and out of the car a half dozen times, this mother's youngest had finally gone to sleep. She had one more errand to run. She knew she shouldn't leave her children in the car, but she admitted being tempted, thinking, "It's only for a moment." She took the children into the market with her, but that feeling of being torn is completely natural. What matters is what we do when we feel that way.

Conflicts like this occur every day:

- The phone rings and you run into the house to answer it, leaving your preschooler in the front yard.

- The washing machine goes off balance and you leave your toddler unattended to adjust it.

- Your first grader has whined incessantly to be left in the toy section while you shop and you give in.

- Your kindergartner wants to walk to school alone and, against your better judgment, you agree.

Lack of adequate supervision is the leading cause of death in the United States. It is a personal safety issue that comes from parental ambivalence, unacknowledged risk-taking, and denial, as much as economics or personal circumstances.

Safety for you and your children is not just a set of rules. It is a series of little decisions. Recognize ambivalence when it occurs. When you recognize it, you can *choose* what to do, rather than letting the situation choose for you.

About Children

Negotiating personal safety decisions with children is complex. **On the one hand, there is the knowledge that your children are vulnerable no matter how careful you are. On the other is the recognition that children simply can't grow up if they aren't allowed, at some point, to move about in the world.**

Personal safety includes teaching rules to your children so they have guidelines and the ability to think on their feet when they're out on their own. It also includes making clear decisions about the limits you will set at various stages in your children's lives.

As obvious as this may seem, children are always stretching for more independence and parents make decisions every day that fail to take into account the reality of the situations in which they place their children. For example, what factors would enter into your decision about the age and circumstances under which you would agree to your child's request to:

- ride a bicycle around the block (i.e., out of sight and hearing distance),

- stay in the car while you run into the store (i.e., out of sight and hearing distance),

- go to the bathroom alone (restaurant, public park, stadium, etc.).

The process of making these decisions is integral to learning to think about personal safety. For example, I had several discussions with a mother whose kindergartner was very independent and demanded to walk to school alone. She could simply have said no, but she wanted to encourage his independence. After discussing the safety issues, she gave him a choice. He could either walk with his mother until they could see the school and then she would watch while he walked the rest of the way alone or she would arrange for him to walk with an older child whose judgment she trusted. This was an agreeable transition that respected her son's needs and kept him safe.

Gradually giving children permission and the ability to do things on their own is part of growing up. But children are not responsible for raising themselves. They cannot be given the ability to make decisions about when they will assume new risks. Adults bear the major responsibility for decisions about the care of children. Adults are responsible for protecting the well-being of children—for keeping them safe. This book was written to help you do that and to help them keep themselves safe when they are alone or when our efforts fail.

The Basics . . .

As parents, we quite naturally avoid the reality that our children may be sexually abused by someone we know. We fear kidnapping by a stranger but don't want to alarm our children or overreact. We downplay the risks, thinking, "I'm safety conscious" or "I never leave my children alone." At the same time, we fear that our children are vulnerable. And we're right.

"Child abuse and neglect in the United States now represent a national emergency. . . . Protection of children from harm is not just an ethical duty; it is a matter of national survival." This call for action from the U.S. Advisory Board on Child Abuse and Neglect has come every year.* Child abuse is what too many children experience every day of their lives.

- Over 3 million cases of child abuse were reported in 1995 in the United States.

- Eighty-five to 90 percent of sexual abuse happens with a person known to the child.

- One in every four girls and one in every six boys will be sexually abused by the age of eighteen.

*Sources for statistics and evaluations cited herein may be found in the Notes on Sources.

- Approximately one-third of sexual abuse cases in-volve children six years of age or younger.

- The Children's Defense Fund estimates that 5.2 mil-lion children age thirteen and under are left without adult supervision each day.

These facts are hard to believe and most people feel they must be exaggerated. But most people who were abused don't talk about it. I remember one PTA board meeting I attended to discuss implementation of the Safe Child Program in the school. After I reported the statistics cited above, one woman said to me, "That just isn't possible. I don't know anyone who was sexually abused as a child." Very quietly, the woman across from her said, "I was." And a moment later, the man beside me followed with "I was, too."

As overwhelming as these statistics are, they do not tell the whole story. Evidence is mounting that child abuse is the precur-sor to many of the major social problems in this culture. Consider these figures:

- Ninety-five percent of child abusers were themselves abused as children.

- Eighty percent of substance abusers were abused as children.

- Eighty percent of runaways cite child abuse as a factor.

- Seventy-eight percent of our prison population were abused as children.

- Ninety-five percent of prostitutes were sexually abused as children.

Not every child who is abused has problems of this magni-tude. But child abuse is destructive. It robs far too many children of their ability to live their lives feeling positive about themselves and being able to become contributing members of our society.

When we recognize how often children are victimized, it brings us directly to the question of what we should do. There are many avenues that can lead to change. Public education, greater community watchfulness and sense of responsibility for the well-being of all children, tougher legislation, more vigorous prosecution, stiffer penalties, and treatment programs for perpetrators are all important.

Schools are increasingly recognizing their role in prevention education. Ninety-two percent of all teachers believe instruction in prevention of child abuse is effective. Parental support of prevention programs in the schools has increased as programs have become more appropriate to the developmental needs and abilities of children. Ninety percent of the public believe that all elementary schools should offer child abuse prevention programming.

Still, most communities have no broad-based and consistent approach to teaching young children the skills they need to reduce their vulnerability to abuse.

Equally important, as parents, we need to know that when all our efforts to protect our children fail and they find themselves alone with a perpetrator, they will have the necessary skills to act effectively and prevent abuse. *The Safe Child Book* and the Safe Child Program provide parents, children, and schools with a unique and powerful approach to accomplishing this end.

Does Prevention Work?

The past decade of research has provided a clear road map for parents and schools seeking to prevent child abuse and abduction.

- It is now evident that "one-shot" efforts, including storybooks, videotapes, games, comics, and plays, alone are not adequate to provide real skill-building for children.

- Developmentally appropriate materials are essential.

- It is compellingly obvious that prevention efforts that begin in second or third grade are already too late, as about half of child abuse begins before that age.

- Preschool appears to be the "most teachable moment" for prevention education to begin.

- Prevention education should be experientially based. Children learn new ideas by watching, listening, and discussion, but skills are learned by doing, by giving children an opportunity to rehearse prevention strategies.

- It is not necessary for programming to be explicit in order to be effective. Fear and anxiety levels are lower with approaches that teach prevention without talking directly about abusive situations.

- The opportunity to apply concepts and turn them into skills through role-play, rehearsing prevention strategies, are at the heart of empowering children to prevent abuse.

This book takes the research and knowledge about child abuse and translates it into specific steps *you and your family* can take to prevent sexual abuse and abduction.

As you read this book, it will be useful to notice what is upsetting to you, what makes you want to stop reading, what seems hard to understand. These can be clues to your own emotions and, perhaps, experiences with sexual abuse. As you teach prevention to your children, your feelings and your ideas will shape

The purpose of this book is to:

- give you a basic understanding of sexual abuse and abduction,

- provide specific personal safety training skills, techniques, and examples to use with your children,

- encourage you to portray the world to your children as a positive place, and

- lessen your anxiety about your children's safety so you can allow them the freedom of movement they need as they grow up.

what you say and do. The more you understand about them, the more effective you can be with your children.

The Safe Child Book is based on the Safe Child Program. After working with children who had experienced abuse and were living with the effects, I developed the Safe Child Program to prevent child abuse in 1981. It has continued to evolve as we learn more about protecting children. The program focuses on prevention of sexual, emotional, and physical abuse, prevention of abuse and abduction by strangers, and safety for children who stay home alone. It is intended to further support the efforts of parents by giving children an opportunity to practice the skills with their peers and to provide ongoing discussion and training as children mature. To date, over a million children and their parents have participated in the program throughout the world.

We know the Safe Child approach is effective from two equally important sources. The first is program evaluation that I discuss throughout this book. The second is anecdotal evidence coming from families whose children have averted abuse or abduction by using the techniques they had learned. In each case, the parents were understandably shaken and their children were calmly saying things like "I don't know why you are upset. You taught me what to do and I did it. Everything is okay now." Developing your children's ability to take care of themselves as a natural part of what they do every day is the intention of this book.

I will suggest some new rules and some changes in the old rules that enable children to be "smart" about their safety without being afraid. My first goal is to provide real protection for your children. The second is to help your children feel safe in the world. The third is to help parents think more concretely about their role in child protection.

Safety Without Fear

Parents can't be on guard every minute. Even parents who think they "never leave their children alone" need to recognize their limited ability to protect their children. You may need to answer the telephone while your child is playing in the yard. You could be in aisle three buying apples while your child dashes to aisle four to look at prizes in the cereal boxes. Children spend time with sitters, other family members, at their friends' houses, and in school. It's impossible for you to be available *all the time* to protect your children.

It is, however, your responsibility to protect your children, and part of that responsibility includes teaching them to protect themselves when they must. **The Safe Child Book will show you how to accomplish this without fostering the idea that the world is an evil place or that the people your children love and trust might hurt them.** It will give you positive, reassuring techniques to address the risks effectively and still allow your children to feel loved and nurtured as they grow up.

Teaching these prevention skills will probably mean looking at what you say and do with them from a new perspective. It may include altering the way you think about their safety, and creating some new rules for your children and for yourself. Your children are changing daily, situations and social conditions are changing daily. Safety is a way of thinking for parents and children, not just a set of rules. This book will help you assess your family's ongoing safety needs.

One of the first things to remember is that scare tactics don't work. They overwhelm and paralyze children instead of reassuring and protecting them. For example, the warning "Don't take candy from strangers because it might be poisoned" conjures up a negative image about the world in which they live. It also doesn't work because children don't understand what you mean. As a result, they either take things from strangers because they think "that nice person wouldn't poison me," or they overreact and won't take anything from anyone.

You teach your children to cross the street without fear. You don't tell them horror stories about children killed by careless drivers in order to make them more cautious on the streets. Instead, you deal with these potentially dangerous situations by giving your children basic rules to follow. We're going to take that same sensible approach.

The Safest Child of All

This personal safety training approach builds upon some simple ideas about the abilities of children:

Children can and must be responsible for their own well-being sometimes. When children find themselves in a situation of risk without an adult available to help them, they must use their own resources to protect themselves. Training sharpens their ability to be responsible for themselves when they need to be.

Children can and should speak up for themselves. What they need is permission to speak up and training to do so effectively and appropriately.

Children as young as three, four, and five are able to generalize, to take the rules and guidelines we give them in one context and apply them to another.

Tickling is a good example. If too much tickling makes your children feel uncomfortable or "funny" inside, they will learn with you that it is all right to say "Stop." In the future, they will be able

The Safe Child Book

to generalize, to transfer that ability to speak up when they are touched in some other way that makes them uncomfortable.

Children are capable of making judgments. They can consider the alternatives and make decisions for themselves.

A good example is the five-year-old who told me about a time she refused to take something out of the oven when asked to by the baby-sitter. She knew that the dish might be too heavy and she'd drop it or too hot and she'd burn herself. She was right.

Another preschooler told me about a time his uncle asked to sleep in his bed with him. He said, "No, my bed's for me, not for big people." No one had ever discussed this possibility with him, he just knew what made sense to him and said no.

> **The best defense your children have against sexual abuse and abduction is:**
>
> - a sense of their own power,
>
> - the ability to assess accurately and handle effectively a wide variety of situations,
>
> - knowing where and how to get help, and
>
> - knowing they will be believed.
>
> Children have a right to be safe without being afraid.
>
> Children who think for themselves are the safest children of all.

3

Prevention Begins Early

Prevention training is a natural part of growing up. Between the ages of two and five, children are developing many capabilities that are consistent with the prevention skills they need to learn. Children older than five already have these abilities and the prevention strategies build upon them. The natural abilities children need to recognize and respect include the following:

Children develop a sense of appropriate and inappropriate touching.

Children learn what kind of touch is common with different groups of people. They expect Mom or Dad to check their teeth after brushing, but it would be unusual to have a store clerk ask to check their teeth. Children usually enjoy hugs and kisses from family members. They respond differently to the same type of affection with someone they know less well or with someone who makes them feel uncomfortable. As soon as children begin to express preferences about touch, they can learn the first steps in prevention.

Children have very clear ideas about what they like and don't like.

Children know very early in life what they like and don't like, and they fully explore their ability to express these feelings during the "terrible twos." They discover that there is "Yes" and there is "No." This is the time to begin teaching them that they have permission to speak up and how to do so. Most children stop being so vocal by about age six. They become more adapted and compliant, but they should be encouraged to continue to express themselves. This doesn't mean they always get their way, but they ought to know we are listening.

Children can recognize and learn to respect their instinct.

Children often "sense" that something is wrong before abuse occurs. When children learn to listen to their "inner voice" and to speak up, they are able to stop abuse before it even begins.

We don't always understand what children say. For example, your children may say to you, "Never, ever let that baby-sitter come back." When you ask, "Why not?" they can't explain or answer you. We know that children sometimes intuitively sense that something is wrong and can't describe what they feel. This is part of your child's natural alarm system. It deserves your respect.

I remember one young girl who had been molested by her grandfather since she was three years old. She talked about the day her grandfather's "bouncing her on his knee" felt different than it had before. She felt confused because he was doing it with her parents in the room and they weren't stopping him. She kept looking at her mom and dad for help, but they were talking and laughing while Grandpa was doing this "funny" thing to her. She thought her mom and dad didn't mind and wouldn't do anything to make it stop. She didn't tell anyone about her continuing abuse until she was twelve.

This is an important story because it makes it so clear that we cannot monitor touch for our children. Instead, we need to use their natural ability to recognize touch that is not okay with them and give them the skills to speak up, make it stop, and then tell us. By taking this approach, we retain comfort in our relationships. We let children be the guides of appropriate and inappropriate touching. We preserve the natural and critically important friendliness and affection of children and families.

There is a difference between affection and abuse, and when touching crosses over from one to the other, children sense the difference. The Safe Child approach to prevention empowers children to identify touch that is not all right with them, for whatever reason, and to stop it effectively and appropriately.

How to Use This Book

This book has been written to help you teach your children to prevent sexual abuse and abduction and to enhance their overall safety. It will describe the problems and some solutions.

Use this book as a resource. Discuss and share it with the other adults in your children's lives, such as teachers, grandparents, baby-sitters, neighbors, and friends. Prevention takes place everywhere, and the more reinforcement your children get from other adults in their lives, the more successful they will be in keeping themselves safe.

Thinking about prevention begins when children are born, but practical applications and teaching your children to take care of themselves begin between two and three years of age. The concepts of personal safety training in this book are applicable to children of all ages. When the rules change or special problems arise for different ages, I will note it for you.

Of the various techniques I suggest, the "What If . . ." game (chapter 4) is one of the most practical and instructive. It is a simple question-and-answer game that helps you and your children look at everyday situations in a new way. In fact, you probably already use it to some degree. For instance, what if the dog chews up this book before you finish it? Although the "What If . . ." questions teach your children about serious issues, they are presented

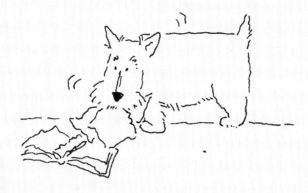

in a light and nonthreatening manner. Use it, enjoy it, adapt it to the places and situations in your own life.

The fundamentals of personal safety training should be taught carefully and thoughtfully, as you would teach swimming, crossing the street, or riding a bicycle. Once mastered, they are skills that can help to keep children safe. As children get older, the rules can change as their needs change. Consistent reinforcement and ongoing discussion about personal safety are the keys to long-term personal safety for your children.

Personal safety training, prevention of abuse, and prevention of abduction are delicate subjects to teach your children, and you may feel that you've made mistakes in dealing with them. Don't be hard on yourself. Just let your children know that you have some new ideas and rules you'd like to discuss with them. Most children are astonishingly receptive to this simple and immediate approach.

Because abuse and abduction generally occur when you're not there to help, one of the most effective things you can do is train your children to protect themselves when you cannot do so. Prevention education at the level of the child begins from what your children know, from what they've already experienced, from the natural abilities I have just described. From there, you build not only self-confidence in their ability to think on their feet and make choices that keep them safe but teach real skills that make them safer.

In addition, when you know—because you've played the games and talked about the rules—that your children can handle themselves in a wide variety of situations, you'll find it is easier for you to let go. When you know your children have the ability to take care of themselves if they need to, you can allow them the freedom of movement they need to be healthy, strong, confident, and safe.

4

The "What If . . ." Game

"What If . . ." is a teaching game that uses your children's sponta-
neous questions as a springboard for discussion. By encouraging
your children to talk about their thoughts, and by discussing your
own reactions and ideas to a "What if . . ." question, you and your
children can agree on a resolution, a strategy for handling it. The
game originates with any questions that begin with "What if. . . ."
It can be played any time, any place, and can cover any subject.

We all use the "What If . . ." game to practice for the things we
can anticipate in life, we just haven't given it a name. "What if my
boss calls me on the carpet at the meeting tomorrow?" "What if
we won the lottery?" "What if I'd hit that rabbit when the children
were in the car?"

The "What If . . ." game will be used to establish your family
rules and to teach all the personal safety skills discussed in this

The purpose for any "What If . . ." game is:

1. to find out what your children think,

2. to talk about possible solutions to a problem,

3. to agree on one solution that seems the best and, from
   that, to establish working guidelines for what you or
   your children would do in such a situation.

book. It is important that you understand the game and how it is played most effectively.

A Window into Your Children's Minds

Children ask "What if . . ." questions that reflect their own fears, concerns, anxieties, and curiosities. Children hear reports of situations experienced by other people that they then apply to themselves. For example, children see the story of a missing or kidnapped child on the news. They translate their reactions into "What if . . ." questions. "What if I had been playing in my yard when that kidnapper came around?" They embellish and modify the details of the story trying to understand. They want to experience some sense of control over the possibility that it could happen to them. Using "What if . . ." questions, they can talk about all the ways they might handle such an event. The game is an opportunity for them to explore ideas, to feel more in control, and to learn real prevention skills.

When children ask "What if . . ." questions, you should resist the urge to answer and let your children answer the "What if . . ." question first. You will discover how they think, what their concerns are, how they solve problems, how they think the world works, and what they know and don't know about keeping themselves safe. Adults answer children's questions, thinking that's why they asked. That isn't always true. When you give children the answers, you deny them an opportunity to confront and resolve their own questions.

By listening instead, you can get accurate information about your children's concerns. They can ask difficult or "silly" questions without feeling embarrassed or foolish. They can talk about their feelings and experiences. Most important of all, your children can use the "What If . . ." game to report an incident they might otherwise keep secret.

Children often don't tell about something that has happened to them because they don't want to upset anyone. In the "What If . . ." game, children can pretend it didn't happen, even though it did. Because it's only a "What If . . . ," it's a bit like make-believe and it is easier to talk about. Your child can find out how you will react and then decide if he or she wants to tell you what happened.

Getting Started

Children can initiate the "What If . . ." by simply asking a question that begins with "What if . . ." I remember a father whose son kept asking, "What if there's no food in the house?" The father replied they'd go to the store. His son then asked, "Well, what if there's no food at the store?" The father's answer generated another question and on and on.

After I discussed the "What If . . ." game with the father, things went very differently. When his son asked, "What if there's no food in the house?," the father responded, "That's a good question. What do you think?" With that opening, the child was able to talk about his real concern. Dad was unemployed and his son wanted to know what they'd do when they ran out of food and money.

Remember, when a "What if . . ." question is asked, don't answer the question yourself, let your children find the answers independently. For example, in response to a younger child's "What if . . . ," you could say something like:

"That's a really good question. What do you think?"

"Gee, I haven't thought about that. What do you think?"

"I have some ideas about that, but I'd like to know what you think first."

For older children, you might respond with:

"I'd like to hear what you think about that."

"I don't know exactly what I'd do. What do you think?"

Some children will balk at going first. If your child wants you to go first, do so. After a few "What If . . ." games, you can begin to take turns and say, "I went first last time."

Remember, it *is* a game. Avoid making an issue over any part of it or the value will be lost. The "What If . . ." game is not a confrontation. It is an opportunity to share ideas and initiate discussion.

The "What If . . ." Game Should Never Frighten

Part of the value of the "What If . . ." game is that parents can introduce situations for discussion in a nonthreatening way. It can help you identify your children's skills and inform your decisions about setting limits and safety rules.

Remember, the idea of the "What If . . ." game is to teach skills without *adding* to the fears and anxieties your children may already have. You should ask "What if . . ." questions that create no *new* fears or anxieties for your children. Start with a "What if . . ." example your children have already expressed. For instance, most children think about getting lost in a shopping center, at a stadium, or in some other crowded place. Using this example is an ideal way to get started.

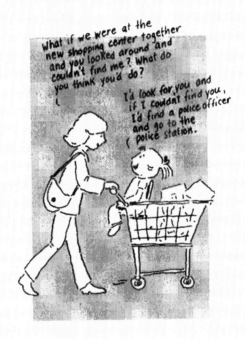

The Safe Child Book

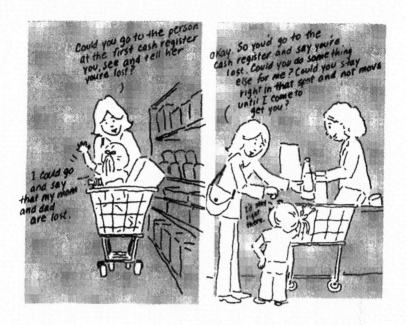

The most enjoyable way to illustrate a "What If . . ." such as this one is to role-play, or act out, the actual situation. You can portray a variety of characters: a cashier, a well-meaning friend or customer, and a "grumpy" store manager. It is important that your children realize that *these are not bad people*, especially the "grumpy" store manager. Your children can play themselves and learn through the role-plays to say no, and to stick to it, even in the face of an adult who seems threatening or physically tries to take them somewhere.

Even when you are pretending to take them away or overpower them, I cannot emphasize strongly enough that your children should never feel frightened or insecure. The game should not be alarming. Play gently, be silly and reassuring. The point is to have them understand the imbalance of power between adults and children and to discover that they have resources for attracting attention that are more effective than just trying to get away.

The "What If . . ." game I have just described sounds as if it is about children getting lost and what they should do. In fact, in teaching this "What If . . . ," you are teaching prevention of abduction. At the same time you're talking about being lost, you're teaching your children what to do and what to say when they are asked to go with, or are being forced to go with, someone. **What's important to note is that you are teaching prevention of abduction without ever mentioning abduction and without producing fear in your children.**

Through the game, your children learn that by anticipating, planning, and acting effectively, a difficult situation can be handled successfully. It is this aspect of the game that makes it the single most valuable tool you have for teaching safety to your children.

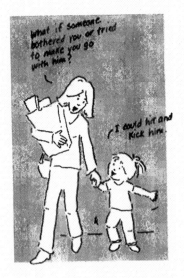
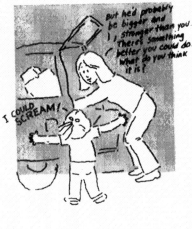

The Safe Child Book

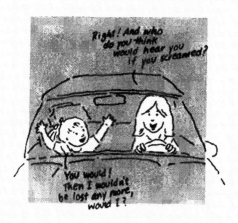

Special Issues for Children of Different Ages

Three- to Six-Year-Olds

Preschoolers and kindergartners play the "What If . . ." game with enthusiasm. The range and diversity of their "What if . . ." questions are astonishing. They are not the carefree spirits we sometimes imagine them to be, but complex people with their own fears and concerns.

Recognizing that your young children think about their own safety is an *opportunity* for you. This is the ideal time for your children to learn that they are capable of making good choices and taking care of themselves and that you want them to do so.

Questions preschoolers might ask include: "What if you didn't come to pick me up and everyone went home?" or "What if my teacher said I could go home with her?" or "What if you fell down and hurt your head?" or "What if someone came to the door when you were in the bathtub?"

Seven- to Nine-Year-Olds

Seven- to nine-year-olds are the most vulnerable group for abuse. They have more freedom to come and go, walking to school, running errands, shopping alone, playing at friends'

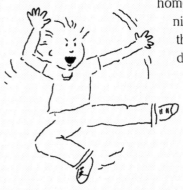

homes, participating in camps and organized sports, etc. At the same time, they often feel insecure about what to do in new situations. Specific preparation through the "What If . . ." game is important to reduce the risk that goes along with their increased freedom.

Children in this age group have the most distorted perceptions about what they can do to solve problems. They sometimes have what I call a "karate mentality." They believe they will "karate chop" their way to safety. While these fantasies are natural and healthy, they should be tempered with a clear distinction between reality and make-believe. This is most easily accomplished by demonstration.

Adults are bigger and stronger. If your children believe they can keep themselves safe by physical power, show them that it's not so. Safety comes from a real understanding of what works and what doesn't work. This is one of the most important distinctions children can learn at this age.

Ten- to Sixteen-Year-Olds

Children ten and up are more easily embarrassed and as they move into adolescence may believe that their parents do not trust them or take them seriously. The "What If . . ." game is particularly important for this group. For example, to check your reactions, your child might ask, "What if I heard that my friend John was invited to join a shoplifting club?" or "What if the other kids got caught smoking in the bathroom and I was there?"

Embarrassment, peer pressure, and a developing sense of independence are the primary factors that keep children ages ten and up from communicating with their parents. These personal pressures can prevent your children from getting out of a dangerous situation. The "What If . . ." game

The Safe Child Book

may seem immature and silly to preteens and adolescents, but it can be revised to make it effective.

Let them take the lead, listen more than you talk, and pay attention to any underlying theme in what they're saying. This is particularly true if the scenario is one step removed by suggesting that it is their friend who wants to know what to do. For example, when your daughter says, "Molly was wondering what she should do if a boy tries to kiss her, but she doesn't want to ask her mom."

Preteens and adolescents don't want to expose their vulnerability, their insecurities, and their attempts to be more grown up. They try to solve situations themselves rather than asking for help. It is essential that families develop a way of handling the increasing conflict between the desire for privacy and independence, and the need to acquire problem-solving skills in adolescence.

When Children Ask Questions Repeatedly

Occasionally children get stuck in a "What if . . ." and repeatedly ask the same question. Usually, the problem is simply that the real question, the source of the child's concern, is not being addressed. When this happens, the "What If . . ." should be broken down into smaller, more workable pieces until you discover the real issue.

The most telling illustration I've had of this problem involved a five-year-old who, after the fire department visited her school, kept asking, "What if there is a fire in the house?" Her mother carefully discussed the safety procedures and drew fire escape routes that were tacked on the walls. It didn't help. The child continued to repeat her question.

When her mother called me, I suggested she ask, "What if there is a fire in the house? What do you think would be the biggest problem?" or "What would be the hardest part?"

A week later, a less frustrated mother reported that her initial question had released a flood of specific questions about what would happen to toys, blankets, schoolbooks, and other treasures

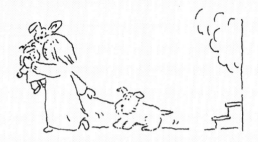

in a fire. They discussed each of these questions and after a few days, her daughter relaxed and the questions stopped. The initial question, "What if there is a fire in the house?," had not been the real question. Only by getting to the real question was the child reassured.

Older children, around nine or ten, tend to stop asking questions if you don't pick up on their underlying concerns. That is why the "What If . . ." game format, in which they talk first, serves the purpose of assuring that you know your child's concern *before* you make your suggestions.

"What If . . ."—Parents Take the Lead

While the "What If . . ." game should be played mostly in response to your children's questions, there are also questions you will want to initiate. When you start a "What If . . ." game, present examples that teach them what to do without producing fear or anxiety.

For example, your children can learn that it's all right for them to say no to anyone without your suggesting that people are bad. The idea can be learned by "silly" questions, but the examples are real enough so that your children learn they can say no. To teach this, you might say:

"What if your teacher said, 'Today we're all going to take our shoes and socks off and go out and play in the snow.'" Children will laugh and say, "Of course I wouldn't. I'd catch a cold."

Or "What if the sitter asked you to go for a ride with her boyfriend?"

When you're thinking of a "What if . . ." question you want to ask your children, ask yourself the question first. If you think the question will create any fear or anxiety for your children, ask it some other way. An *inappropriate* question might sound like this: "What if someone came and snatched your baby sister out of the front yard when you were taking care of her? What would you do?" This type of "What if . . ." creates a new fear rather than teaching prevention. It would be better to ask, "What if you were in the yard with your baby sister and someone you didn't know came into the yard? What would you do?"

Asking "What if . . ." questions that are *too* specific can be misleading and it doesn't allow the children to extend the example to other occurrences. They teach children to watch out only for that particular set of circumstances. Using general examples allows for expansion to include any situation and creates no new fear.

We don't have the right to project our own fears onto our children. It is always possible to ask your question in a way that is fun and instructive and children can and do generalize from it. If you know the skill you want to teach, ask a general "What if . . ." that has no specific details or descriptions. This will allow you to determine whether your children can handle the type of situation about which you are concerned.

When the "What If . . ." game becomes a regular part of your family's discussions, your children can talk about fears and anxieties as they come up, rather than privately worrying about them. For example, there was a six-year-old abducted from a playground outside Denver. Her death, and the ensuing media coverage, created enormous anxiety for all the schoolchildren in the area. This was a perfect time to use the "What If . . ." game to talk about what children could do if someone approached them.

Never respond to a "What if . . ." by saying, "Oh, that will never happen to you." When you say this, your children hear, "Mom and Dad don't want to talk about it," which only

DON'T	DO
"What if you were walking home from school and a big white van pulled up and a man wearing a cowboy hat tried to make you get into his car?"	"What if you were walking home from school and you saw a car or person who seemed suspicious or that you felt funny about?"
This is teaching the child to watch out for white cars and cowboy hats.	This is not frightening or so detailed that the child can visualize a specific danger. It teaches the general skill that can be applied as needed.
"What if your baby-sitter asked you to take down your pants and let him touch your penis?"	"What if your baby-sitter touched you in a way you didn't like?"
This creates an idea your child has never thought of and the anxiety that goes along with it.	This generic question allows you to talk about the idea without giving your child more information than he needs.
"What if someone broke a window and came into your bedroom with a gun when you were home alone?"	"What if you were home by yourself and you thought you heard a noise?"
This is a frightening possibility. Expect nightmares if you ask "What if . . ." questions like this.	This is something that happens to all of us. You can discuss options without alarm.

The Safe Child Book

increases their anxiety. Instead of dismissing the question, recognize it as an opportunity to discuss their concern.

One Essential "What If . . ." Question

What if children misbehave and something bad happens? What do they do? They often don't tell anyone. For example, if they go to someone's house without permission and are sexually abused, they may not tell because they broke the rules. It is imperative that your children have a way to talk to you if something happens, even when they feel guilty.

Children almost always feel that they are at fault when something bad happens. If they were misbehaving, they believe that is why something bad happened. Even if they weren't doing anything wrong, they think they were.

Children learn this from us. When we say, "Well, if you hadn't been riding your bike so fast, you wouldn't have fallen off and cut your leg," we are telling children that getting hurt is a function of their own mistakes. This belief will prevent them from telling us they have been abused or hurt because they will be certain they did something to cause or deserve it.

Children are egocentric and think they cause just about everything. Guilt is a natural response to injury or abuse. At the same time, it is important to balance this point of view by talking with children about bad things that happen over which they have no control.

One easy way to do this is to ask, "Did you feel it was your fault?" when something painful or sad happens. Cut knees, broken toys, and pets that die are all opportunities to talk about your child's sense of guilt or blame and to counterbalance that with a discussion about the many things that happen to all of us that are simple accidents or are beyond our control.

At other times, children don't tell because they aren't certain what will happen if they do. To help your children tell you about things that happen to them when they've broken the rules, they must know what they can expect from you. The following "What if . . ." should help:

"What if you go somewhere we've told you never to go or you go with someone we've told you never to go with and something bad happens or you get into a lot of trouble. How will you tell me?"

Whatever their response, follow with: "If something like that happened, we'd want to know because we love you and want you to be safe." Follow up with: "We'd take care of the bad thing that happened and you could decide what should happen because you broke the rules." (In a real situation, they'll be a lot tougher on themselves than you'll ever be.)

It is important that consequences for children's misbehavior under these circumstances be imposed. Otherwise, they make the mistake of thinking that the bad thing that happened to them was their punishment. The consequences for their misbehavior should be natural or logical, that is, they should have something to do with the misbehavior. They should be set without anger, and your child should feel that he or she learned something from what happened.

"What If . . ." Checklist

- Always play the game with a nonthreatening "What if . . ."

- Use role-playing or acting out the story as a way to make the game more fun and to establish the expected behavior.

- Never respond to your children's "What if . . ." by saying, "Oh, don't worry about that. That will never happen to you."

- Your children should ask most of the "What if . . ." questions.

- You should not ask questions that alarm or frighten your children.

- Be aware of age differences when playing the "What If . . ." game so older children aren't insulted or turned off.

- If your children keep asking the same thing over and over, that isn't the question they want answered.

- Make sure your children know in advance how to tell you about something that has happened following misbehavior or breaking the rules.

5

Understanding Sexual Abuse

As much as we try to protect and care for our children, we simply are not present to prevent sexual abuse. Prevention means preparing your children to prevent abuse, to stop an assault at its inception. Training gives your children the ability to do that, even with someone who is older, more knowledgeable, more powerful, and, even, loved by them. Prevention training tells them what they need to know, gives them the skills to act, and assures them that you will believe and help them if something happens.

Prevention of sexual abuse can be taught without talking about sexual abuse. Children don't need to be told what sexual abuse is, who perpetrators are, how they operate, what they do or why. Children don't need a list of ways in which they might be abused. They need to acquire the ability to make decisions for themselves based on what they believe to be true at that moment. They need permission to speak up. They need specific techniques to stop what's being done to them. And they must know they will be believed and supported by the adults in their lives.

Parents, on the other hand, do need to understand the nature of sexual abuse. The prevention techniques are based on the patterns and methods used by the 85 to 90 percent of abusers who know and have a relationship with the child. The more you know about what sexual abuse is, who abuses children, how they operate, and why children become involved, the more effectively you can teach prevention to your children.

What Is Sexual Abuse?

Sexual abuse is legally defined as any sexual contact with a child or the use of a child for the sexual gratification of someone else. It includes exhibitionism, child pornography, fondling of the genitals or asking the child to do so, oral sex, and attempts to penetrate the vagina or anus. Fondling is the most common form of sexual abuse.

The insidious and sordid nature of child sexual abuse cases is overwhelming, even for those of us who see it daily. **While the spectacular cases are the ones we read about, most sexual abuse is quietly occurring, with no physical injury or life-threatening acts, between the child and someone he or she trusts.** It is this "quiet" aspect of sexual abuse that makes it so hard to recognize, so hard to believe, and so hard to accept.

Why Sexual Abuse Is So Destructive

The physical things that happen to children who are sexually abused are damaging about 10 percent of the time. The greatest long-term injury to children, however, comes from their sense of betrayal by the person who abused them. The more important the

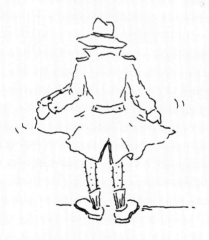

relationship, the bigger the betrayal and loss, especially when the abuse occurs with a parent or grandparent. This betrayal is compounded if the child tells and is not believed or the abuse is not stopped.

Sexually abused children feel a loss of control; they feel victimized and uncertain about whom to trust. This emotional damage is far more long-lasting than the physical effects and requires careful, nurturing support and counseling to repair.

Who Are the Perpetrators?

"Pedophilia" is the term for sexual preference for children. It has nothing to do with homosexuality. Some pedophiles prefer girls, some prefer boys, and some have no preference. Eighty-five to 90 percent of all sexual abuse takes place with someone the child knows and trusts. In 1981, David Finkelhor, a leading researcher in this field, reported that 30 percent of sexual abuse takes place with a family member, including parents, grandparents, siblings, aunts, uncles, and stepparents. While most pedophiles are men, his research shows that at least 20 percent of all perpetrators are female.

Sexual abusers are generally people who were abused as children. They are people who were victimized and who continue the cycle of abuse by victimizing others. For those who become perpetrators, sexual abuse of children is a way of life. The United States Justice Department reports that they assault an average of more than seventy children in their "career" of offending. Some abuse hundreds of children.

Those perpetrators who abuse children they know are seeking an intimate, nonjudgmental, affectionate relationship with a child. **They need to exercise power and control over children and to believe that children "willingly" enter, if not initiate and encourage, the sexual relationship.** They rarely acknowledge that what they are doing "hurts" children.

There is no profile that I can give you to help you identify potential abusers. They tend to be people we like and trust and their obvious and genuine care for children earns them our admiration. This, in part, explains why it is so hard for us to accept it when we have trusted a perpetrator and how difficult it is for children to tell us what happened.

Incest

This is unquestionably the most difficult part of sexual abuse for parents to think about. Unless you have experienced it, it is unthinkable that someone who is a part of your family would violate your child's trust and love in this way. Nevertheless, Diana Russell, in one of the most comprehensive studies to date, found that 16 percent of the women participating in her study had experienced sexual abuse by a family member who was at least five years older than they were. Father/daughter incest was reported by 4.5 percent of the women.

The prevention techniques described in *The Safe Child Book* are designed to prevent incest as well as abuse by other people known to the child. It is not appropriate to suggest to children that the members of their family would sexually abuse them. As a parent, however, you should know that you will be teaching techniques to prevent both.

Stepparents as Abusers

Diana Russell, also in her 1981 report, confirms that stepfathers are much more likely to sexually abuse their stepdaughters than biological fathers. This is a very difficult problem. You can't begin a new relationship suspecting abuse. At the same time, you can't ignore the risks. Using these prevention techniques is a good medium ground.

Boyfriends and stepfathers have a powerful edge with children. They know that children want their moms to be happy, and

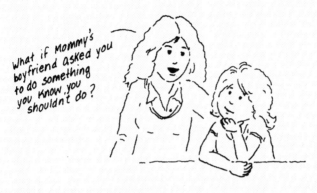

What if Mommy's boyfriend asked you to do something you know you shouldn't do?

these abusers will tell children that they will go away if the child isn't cooperative. They point out how unhappy that would make Mom, and children go along rather than create upheaval. They don't want to be responsible for Mom's relationship breaking up.

Reducing children's vulnerability is accomplished by talking to your children about what they should do if your boyfriend or their stepfather asks them to do something they know they shouldn't do. Talk about the difference between respect and blind obedience. Let your children know that you will never stop loving them. Tell them that they can always come to you if they are uncomfortable with something being said to them or done to them by someone else. In teaching the prevention techniques described in *The Safe Child Book*, be sure your children know they apply to everyone.

Do Children Abuse One Another?

I get a lot of calls from parents who wonder if their children have been sexually abused by a playmate or a sibling. When children are abused, they may reenact with other children what happened to them. This sexual activity is both inappropriate and confusing. It requires reeducation of the children so they can find more appropriate ways to play with one another as well as therapeutic intervention with the initiating child.

In addition, every effort should be made to discover the perpetrator who sexually abused the first child. This may be another child. If so, find out who abused that child. Follow the chain of abuse. There is always an older perpetrator at the end. Once again, reeducation for all the affected children is needed, as well as increased supervision until the behavior is no longer an issue.

The Tools of the Child Abuser

Friendship, trust, and bribery are the most common and effective tools of abusers. They take the time to get to know children and to develop relationships with them. At some point, they initiate what perpetrators call the "grooming process"—they "test" to see if this is a child who can be abused. For example, they might stick their hand up the child's shirt while tickling or wrestling. They might ask the child to sit close to them while riding in the car and rest their hand on his or her inner thigh. These are not inherently abusive activities, but they do test a child's ability to be assertive in a situation that is uncomfortable.

When a child resists, perpetrators often respond with: "Don't you like me?" "Don't you love me?" "Don't you want to be my friend?" In effect, they are using their relationship with the child to obtain his or her compliance. This, combined with the abuser's greater power, knowledge, and experience, tips the balance against the child, and most give in. If, on the other hand, a child has learned prevention skills and is firm about stopping the behavior, the perpetrator generally will move on to another, less resistant child.

Why Children Let It Continue

Being smaller and more trusting, children often accept the assurances of their "friend" and allow the uncomfortable activity to continue. This encourages the perpetrator and the activity quickly escalates until it becomes sexual abuse. Once this happens, it is very difficult for children to extricate themselves. The four primary reasons children don't tell are:

1. *Guilt.* This always accompanies sexual abuse. Children say to themselves, "If something bad happened to my body and I didn't stop it, then *I* must be bad or it must be my fault. And it happened with someone I liked a lot."

2. *Relationship.* In spite of the abuse, children continue to value the relationship with the perpetrator. They realize the relationship will end if they tell about the abuse. This is a powerful concern and should not be forgotten after the abuse is discovered. Many children, and even parents, continue to feel protective toward the abuser after the abuse has been revealed, especially if the perpetrator is a family member.

3. *Fear.* Children are afraid they won't be believed if they tell someone. This is very real, particularly when the offender is someone loved and trusted by the family or the community. Children also may be afraid that someone will be hurt if they tell. They may believe that they are protecting other children in the family by allowing the abuse to continue.

4. *Disruption.* Children recognize that telling will create family upheaval, possible divorce, court appearances, jail, etc. In letting the abuse continue, children may feel they are protecting the ones they love.

Do Children Lie About Sexual Abuse?

Almost without exception, children do not lie about sexual abuse, except to deny that it happened. If a child can tell you what happened, you must believe that it did occur. This does not mean that children may not misinterpret or misreport an event. Because young children don't generally have access to explicit sexual information, they don't "make up" or "fantasize" sexual

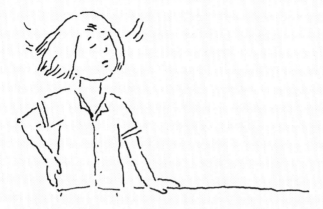

abuse. Children who can talk about their abuse in detail have experienced it.

As children learn more about sexual abuse—particularly from the media—parents and professionals are concerned that false reports will increase, especially with preadolescents and adolescents. While this is a possibility, the child who is fabricating reports of sexual abuse can be unmasked quickly by an experienced interviewer. Current studies indicate fewer than 1 percent of child abuse reports are false.

Children more often tell us without meaning to. For example, if you see your children "playing sex" (not playing doctor), if you get a "French kiss" good-night, if you suddenly hear new names for body parts or see sexually provocative behavior, no matter how alarmed or upset you feel, you should calmly ask, "Who taught you that?" or "Who else plays that game with you?" **Any time a child can answer these questions and talk about a sexual abuse experience, you must believe it happened, even if they get scared and tell you a few hours later that they made it up.**

Sexual Abuse and Sex Education

Training in the prevention of sexual abuse is not the same as sex education. I do believe, however, that understanding his or her body is important to a child's positive self-image, and it can help reduce his or her vulnerability to exploitation and abuse.

It is important to use accurate names for body parts as a way of teaching healthy respect for our bodies. It is customary in our society to use pet names or nicknames for the genitalia. This may be Victorian, or it may be an attempt by parents to "protect" their children's innocence, or it may be a simple continuation of how our parents taught us. Whatever the reason, we don't nickname our eyes or ears or toes, and we should not do it with other body parts, either.

Children who think there is something "secret" or "different" about their genital area are more vulnerable to suggestions that they are "bad" for very normal kinds of play, such as masturbation. This suggestion of "badness" can be a powerful weapon in the hands of a perpetrator. Being comfortable and at ease with their bodies is a simple and natural beginning for prevention training for children.

Playing Doctor

Observing sexual play is one of the common ways we discover sexual abuse in young children. Normal playing doctor is mutual and healthy exploration and play. It never includes one child victimizing another, nor does it include oral-genital contact or attempts to penetrate the vagina or anus. If you come across suspicious play, simply ask, as I suggested earlier, "What game are you playing?" "Who else plays this game with you?" "How do you play this game?" Children will often tell us exactly where they learned this "game" and we immediately find out if there is a problem.

In all events, it is essential that you not overreact in such a situation. Most children play doctor at some time. If that's the situation you've come upon, use it as an opportunity to initiate discussion and give guidelines. Children want to know about themselves and others. During the preschool years, especially when children are open, if not matter-of-fact, about their bodies, answer their questions. You can also acknowledge that it feels good to touch themselves and that it's all right to do so in private. It is not okay to touch others or ask them to touch you.

Masturbation

Touching the genitals and masturbating are natural parts of growing up. When children begin to play with their genitals in your presence, you might say, "I know it feels good to play with your penis, but it's something that you should do in private, in your own room or the bathroom, not in front of other people." Later, you can add the messages found in the next chapter to teach prevention.

Prevention of Sexual Abuse

In the next chapter, we will use what we know about children, perpetrators, and child abuse to teach prevention skills.

6

Preventing Sexual Abuse

Training in prevention of sexual abuse begins with children's natural abilities, what they already know, and the experiences they've already had. It builds on the following ideas:

Your Body Belongs to You

Children learn they have control over what happens to their bodies when we teach them, and when we show them by our own behavior, that their bodies belong to them.

The first step in prevention is to say to your children:

"Your body belongs to you. You have a right to say who touches you and how. If someone touches you

- in a way you don't like,

- in a way that feels funny or uncomfortable,

- in a way you think is wrong, or

- in a way that your mom or dad would think is wrong, it's okay to say 'No, stop it.'

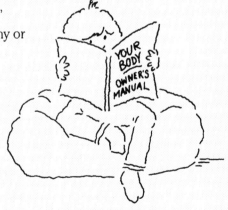

The person should stop."

Illustrate this by recalling times when your children were touched in ways they didn't like or felt uncomfortable about:

- When Aunt Sally pinches their cheeks.

- When next-door neighbor Fred throws them over his head.

- When big sister tickles and won't stop.

- When a friend of Dad's hugs too hard.

None of these examples constitutes sexual abuse. However, when children learn to say no to someone who pinches their cheek, or picks them up, they learn to say no to more intrusive harmful touching. What's new is that it's okay to say NO.

Many children tell me that their bodies belong to God. I suggest to them that they are partners with God. Children help God to take care of them by taking care of their bodies, brushing their hair, dressing themselves, and keeping themselves safe.

Basic Principles of Prevention

- Your body belongs to you.

- You have a right to say who touches you and how.

- If someone touches you in a way you don't like, in a way that makes you feel funny or uncomfortable inside, in a way that you think is wrong, or in a way your mom or dad would think is wrong, it's okay to say no.

- If the person doesn't stop, say, "I'm going to tell," and then tell, no matter what.

- If you're asked to keep a secret, say, "No, I'm going to tell."

Permission to Say No

Your children already know what they like and what they don't like. You are giving them permission to be assertive and teaching them how to speak up—in a way that is acceptable to both of you. Help your children find the words and then practice. They should be able to say them, without hesitation, in a clear, audible voice. Give them many ways to say NO.

"Please stop. I don't like that."

"That's not fun anymore, and I don't want you to do it."

"Leave me alone."

"You shouldn't be asking me to do that. Leave me alone."

"I'm not allowed to do things like that. Please take me home now."

Or simply "Stop."

Verbal messages alone are not enough. Your children also must show with their bodies what they want to say. I often have children in my classes who are saying, "Don't hug me so hard," as they are climbing up on my lap. Children should learn to say no with their bodies at the same time they are saying no with their words.

Private Parts

Many prevention programs teach children that they shouldn't let anyone touch their private parts. This is problematic for several reasons. First, it is a way to avoid talking about what we're talking about. It results in confused children.

One day, my son came home and told me he knew a boy who had seen a girl's private parts. He couldn't say who the boy or girl was. The next day, he told me again that he knew a boy who had seen a girl's private parts. Then he paused and asked me, "What's a private part?" My son knows all the names for genitalia and had never encountered the euphemism "private parts." When children are told not to let anyone touch their private parts as a way to

avoid talking about penises and vaginas, they aren't protected because they have no idea what we are talking about.

Second, most abusers don't begin their abuse with the private parts. They develop the relationship and go through the grooming process as discussed in the previous chapter. By the time perpetrators get to the private parts, it is too late for prevention.

Private parts include the genital area, the buttocks, and the breasts. While it may be tempting for parents to say something like "The parts of your body that your bathing suit and underwear cover up are special parts of your body and no one should touch them," it's preferable to identify the vagina, penis, testicles, buttocks, and breasts.

As children take an interest in their own genitalia, you will gradually want to communicate the following: "You can touch yourself there when you're alone in your bedroom or the bathroom, but other people shouldn't touch you there. Those parts of the body are special for other people, too, and it's not okay for someone older than you to touch you or to ask you to touch their private parts, especially if they ask you to keep it a secret. Exceptions would include times when you're sick or at the doctor, but even then you should tell Mommy and Daddy if you feel uncomfortable about what is happening."

Double Messages

One of the beauties of this approach to prevention is that we don't have to worry about monitoring touch. Rather, we're giving children permission to determine their own comfort or discomfort level with touch and the ability to communicate their wishes effectively.

What is a greater concern for adults is mixed messages. Can you identify how the messages in the following scenarios might be inconsistent with the prevention techniques in this book?

- You're in the grocery store with your preschooler and a friend approaches. Your child immediately goes behind your legs. You urge him to come out and talk to your friend.

- Gram and Gramp come over for dinner. When they're leaving, they want a kiss. Your child says no. You suggest that Gram and Gramp drove a long way, or Gram and Gramp love her very much, or Gram and Gramp might not come next week if they don't get a kiss.

- You want a good-night kiss. Your child says no. You ask, "Don't you love me?" or "Are you mad at me?"

- A friend of the family has hugs and kisses for everyone after a long vacation. Your child resists and your response is "You know we haven't seen her for a long time. You don't want to hurt her feelings."

In all these situations, what we're saying to children is that adults' feelings are more important than their own, that children should suppress their own feelings to please adults. If they don't, they're not being "good" children. Even if the message is unintended, it is what children hear.

The Safe Child Book

This kind of hidden message is very similar to what perpetrators say when children resist sexual abuse. As a result, children give in. Because of the way children interpret our words and actions, they are ill equipped to know that it is absolutely all right to say no and to stick to it no matter what emotional ploys are used to change their minds.

How Should Adults Respond?

When children express uneasiness about any kind of touch, say, "Thank you for telling me you don't like that. I'll try to remember" or "You know, grown-ups can't read your mind. I'm glad you told me to stop" or "It's okay to say no, even if I'm a grown-up."

Note that we aren't labeling any behavior or touch as "good" touch or "bad" touch. We don't want to create any controversy about touching or to confuse children by categorizing touch. We are simply leaving decisions about touching up to them.

More and more, I'm hearing fathers express uncertainty about how they should play with their children, how they should express affection. All the publicity about child abuse has made them almost fearful about touching their own children. The answer is: *just as you always have,* adding only an awareness of the need to be responsive and to reinforce your child's expression of his or her likes and dislikes.

One father described the day he was at the pool with his three-year-old daughter. Her shrieks of delight were misinterpreted by several people who thought she was protesting. He stopped playing with her, but he was also angry that his relationship with her was changed by the opinions and misinterpretations of others.

Prevention does not mean you need to stop touching. Children need all the love, affection, and nurturing you can give them. One of the worst possible consequences of prevention training would be the withdrawal of normal adult affection and play with children. The Safe Child approach to prevention allows children to decide about touching for themselves and gives them permission and support to speak up for themselves.

Three- to Six-Year-Olds

Young children tell me that some of the things they don't like are: kisses on the mouth, getting their shirts tucked in by grown-ups, being picked up, having their hair stroked, having to kiss Grandma and Grandpa or Mom and Dad's friends. All of these are contacts or touching that adults take for granted.

For children, they are sometimes okay, other times they can be unwanted touching, just as sexual abuse is unwanted touching. Respecting children's preferences about all forms of touching, giving them permission to speak up, and developing the skills to speak up effectively all form the foundation for prevention of sexual abuse.

One class of preschoolers demonstrated this brilliantly. I had just completed an exercise with a little girl who said she didn't like to be kissed on the lips. She decided what she would say to her mom and sat down. As she did, a little boy in the group stood up, looked for his mom in the back of the room and said, "Mom, I really love you, but I don't want to be kissed on the lips anymore. I want to be kissed on the cheek." He already knew he didn't like to be kissed on the lips. The class had given him the permission and the words to say so. He wasn't passing up the opportunity.

After your children begin to understand that you are giving them permission to speak up about touching, add, "If someone tries to touch your body, or asks you to touch theirs, you can say no. If someone wants you to do things that you don't do with anyone else, don't let them. If anyone wants you to keep touching a secret, come and tell me."

Seven- to Sixteen-Year-Olds

As children get older, increasingly complex emotions affect their relationships. Peer pressure, the need for approval and acceptance, and embarrassment all become more important. Offenders know this, and skillfully manipulate and exploit these emotions. The following examples can help you teach your school-age children to confront and deal with emotionally complex situations.

"What if your teacher always puts her arm around you when you come up to the front of the room and you like it? But today is different because you missed almost all the words on your spelling test and you're upset. So when she puts her arm around you, you pull away. She pulls you closer. You pull away again and say, 'Leave me alone.' She doesn't understand and says, 'What's bugging you?' loud enough for the kids to hear. How do you feel? What do you do?"

Suggestion: "I missed most of the words on my spelling test. I'm crabby and don't want you to put your arm around me."

"What if your dad's still giving you big bear hugs, but your breasts are developing and his bear hugs are embarrassing and they hurt. How do you tell him?"

Suggestion: "Mom might talk to Dad for you, to let him know you still love him, but bear hugs are out for a while."

"What if your soccer coach hits you on the arm every time he gets near you on the field? The other guys don't seem to mind, but you hate it and ask him to stop. The next day, he does it again. You

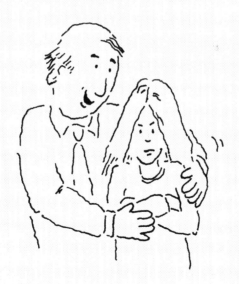

turn to him and tell him to keep his hands to himself. His response is 'You don't like it, get off the team.' What do you do?" (Most children will solve this problem by getting off the team, which is not right, because the problem is with the coach, not with the child.)

"What if you decide to tell your dad? When you do, your dad asks what you did that caused the coach to hit you. When you say, 'Nothing,' your dad says the coach wouldn't hit you for nothing. So you show your dad how he hits you. Then your dad responds with 'Oh, that's part of being on the team and it means the coach likes you.'

"Did Dad understand your problem? Now what do you do? How about telling your mom or your uncle and get help talking to your dad? Just because 'everyone does it' doesn't mean you have to go along."

Remember, none of these examples involves sexual abuse, but they are situations that are hard to handle and give your children practice in applying prevention skills.

We want to teach children to *keep talking,* keep telling until someone listens, understands their problem, and helps. You should use the "What If . . ." game to reinforce and practice getting help for a problem even when it seems no one is listening.

I'm Going to Tell

"I'm going to tell" is one of the most important ways for children to extricate themselves from difficult situations and to avoid a sexual assault. Most perpetrators are known to the child. Seeming compliance by the child is important to them. Children who refuse to go along and who intend to tell are less likely to be victimized.

To review: Your children need to be taught to say, "I don't like that" or "Stop it" or "Leave me alone" or some variation of no any time they're being touched in a way that's not okay with them. They should learn to say, "I'm going to tell if you don't leave me alone" if their first request is ignored. Rather than risk being found out, perpetrators

The Safe Child Book

who are known to the child usually back off when their efforts to persuade the child prove futile.

Parents often ask me, "If my child says no, is he more likely to get hurt?" Usually not. Remember, abusers are looking for a warm, nonjudgmental, affectionate relationship. They don't want to be rejected. Discovery is a greater risk if the perpetrator hurts the child. It's safer and easier for them to walk away, to find another child who will be more compliant. In all cases, children must learn that it's all right to tell what happened to them, even if they promised the abuser they wouldn't tell.

Children also need to learn to tell their parents or someone they trust *any time* they have to say, "I'm going to tell" in order to get someone to stop touching them. And they must know that they will be believed and supported.

Tattling

Children often confuse "I'm going to tell" with tattling. *Tattling is telling on someone the same age as you, or a brother or sister, so you can get them in trouble.* When your children smile at this definition, you'll know they know exactly what you mean.

Telling because they need help with a problem or because a friend needs help or because someone older is bugging them is *never* tattling. This is an easy and clear distinction for children to make when you give them a few examples.

"What if Bobby's big brother was beating up on him, would it be tattling for you to tell me about it?"

No, because Bobby needs help.

"What if someone at your school was stealing your lunch money, would it be tattling to tell your teacher about it?"

No, because that's a problem you need help to solve.

"What if the baby-sitter's boyfriend came over when I wasn't home? He made you promise not to tell. Would it be tattling to tell me?"

No, because someone older is trying to involve you in something they shouldn't be doing.

Remember, the "What If . . ." game is your best tool for practicing and applying the prevention skills.

Preventing Emotional Coercion

Abusers respond to "I'm going to tell" in a variety of ways. If you make your children aware of these ploys before anything happens, perpetrators will have less power and your children will be less vulnerable to abuse.

Bribery. "What if the person who is bugging you says, 'Oh, I'm sorry, I didn't mean to upset you. Let's go get some ice cream and cake.'"

That's bribery. We tend not to talk about bribery with children (perhaps because we use it). But your children need to know that the harder someone tries to get them to keep quiet about something, the more important it is to tell.

I don't care. "What if you say, 'Leave me alone or I'm going to tell,' and the other person says, 'Go ahead and tell. I don't care.'"

When children hear this, they think no one will care. They need to know that you care about them and they should come and tell you about what happened.

No one will believe you. "What if the person says, 'Go ahead and tell, no one will believe you.'"

Children tend to think this anyway. Your children should know that any time they're not believed or not listened to, they should find someone else who will listen and who will help them.

Threats. "What if the person says, 'If you tell, your mom and dad won't love you anymore' or 'If you tell, I'll do something to your dog, or to your baby brother or sister or your mom or dad' or 'I will hurt you or someone you care about if you tell.'"

The message children need to hear from us is: "This is a bigger problem than you can handle. You need to tell someone who can help." Or for younger children: "That's not a real friend. You need to come and tell me about what happened so I can help take care of you. Don't be afraid to tell me. I'm a grown-up and I can help no matter what that other person says."

The Safe Child Book

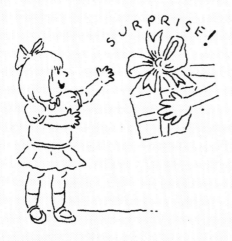

No More Secrets

The No More Secrets Rule is an agreement you make with your family that you won't keep secrets anymore (not even in the family), and if they are asked to keep a secret, your children will say, "No, we don't keep secrets in our family and I'm going to tell." Younger children can simply say, "No, I'm going to tell."

Surprises are okay. Surprises are things that make people happy that get told sooner or later. Secrets are never told. Children quickly learn the difference, and by age four can respond to a request for secrecy about a birthday gift with "That's not a secret, it's a surprise."

Since 85 to 90 percent of perpetrators are known to the child, it's clear that sexual abuse cannot take place without secrecy. Therefore, one of the first things perpetrators will do is find out if the child can keep a secret. If a child steadfastly refuses, most abusers will not risk moving ahead.

Children and Secrecy

Secrecy is often confused with whispering for young children. Explain to them that telling something you only want one person to hear is different from keeping a secret. A secret is when they promise not to tell anyone else.

By age five or six, children can learn that there are many ways to be asked to keep a secret. They enjoy making a game of trying to trick Mom and Dad into keeping a secret without using the word "secret." For example, what if someone says: "This is just between you and me." "Do you promise not to tell anyone else?" "You don't need to tell your mom and dad. I'll tell them later." "We won't tell them about our little game." Your children should respond to all of these requests by saying, "No, I don't keep secrets and I'm going to tell."

By age seven or eight, secrecy is such an integral part of children's lives with their friends that they are reluctant to give it up. This includes friendship clubs, secret bonds, oaths, and pacts.

At this age, the No More Secrets Rule can be narrowed. If a request for secrecy, whether or not the word "secret" is used, seems confusing or odd or uncomfortable, children should refuse. Any effort to keep affection or touching a secret should be firmly refused. Since embarrassment or seeming babyish is increasingly a concern for older children, they might want to say, "I don't like keeping secrets and I don't want to start now" or "I don't like this idea, let's do something else" or "I'd like to go home now."

Privacy is not the same as secrecy. Privacy means you can be by yourself or keep something to yourself. Secrecy means you're bound not to tell. Privacy respects individual needs. Secrecy creates shame in sexual abuse. It's important that children know the difference.

It is the *request* for secrecy that is important. Touching should never have to be a secret and your children should tell any time someone tries to make touching a secret.

Adults Have Rules, Too

Children often get drawn into sexual abuse situations because they trust and love the abuser. They don't realize that adults have rules, too. One of those is: *Adults aren't allowed to ask children to do grown-up things.*

The belief that adults are always in the right can interfere with a child's ability to listen to his or her own inner voice.

Children should know that adults have problems and that they make mistakes. Even if the adult says that the activity is okay, because they have a "special" relationship, children need to be prepared to say no and to tell someone about what happened. Any time an adult asks a child to do something children don't usually do, the child should say no and talk to an adult about what happened.

Whom Do You Tell?

Tell your children that you want to hear about what is happening to them. Parents don't always listen very well and children don't always communicate very well, but they should know it's okay to keep trying until we understand what it is they want to say.

Telling should be like a reflex. Your children should feel that they can *always* tell you, or someone else they trust, what's happened to them. This reflex is instilled through previous experience and constant positive reinforcement. Each time we listen, we teach our children that their feelings and questions are important and will be taken seriously.

Never tell your children whom they can trust. An abuser can be anyone. Children need to make their own decisions about whom they trust. This was illustrated with one child who told me about her uncle. He had been abusing her for two years and she hadn't told anyone because her mother had said to her, "If anything ever happens to me, your uncle will take care of you. He loves all of us and you can always go to him with a problem." When her uncle was the problem, the child didn't know what to do and she was sure her mother wouldn't believe her.

Because children are ambivalent about telling or are afraid to tell, they often tell us in obscure ways that we don't understand. This is not necessarily anyone's fault, but it happens all the time. **For this reason, it is important to teach children to keep**

telling until someone hears them and helps with their problem.

One of the common patterns in incest cases is that of a child who tells someone about the incest at about age six or seven. If that person doesn't listen or help, the child doesn't tell anyone else until about age twelve or thirteen, when he or she is as likely to run away as to tell again.

Children need to know that adults have their own problems and worries, that they don't always listen well and sometimes they can't help. When children ask for help and don't get it, they need to know whom else they can go to. For example, you might say to your children: "What if you had a problem and I was sick? Who would you talk to?" "What if Dad wasn't interested in listening because he was taking care of me, then who could you tell?" "What if the next-door neighbor was out of town?" "What if your teacher was grumpy that day and didn't have time to stop and talk?"

By asking a series of questions, your children can develop a list of people who care about them, who could help them. With problems as complex as sexual abuse, it is important to equip children ahead of time to get help when they can't talk to you.

Identifying Strangers

Teaching parents and children how to deal with strangers is essential for two reasons. First, to give children and parents good skills to prevent abduction. Second, to address the anxiety created for parents and children alike at the thought of stranger abduction.

Stranger Danger programs have been taught for decades. Still, all the evidence shows that children go willingly with strangers. Why? Because children don't hear what adults think they are saying.

Reducing children's vulnerability requires that parents and children have basic information about stranger offenders and how they behave. It includes understanding what children believe about strangers and how that makes them more vulnerable. This chapter will help parents and children develop specific ground rules to enhance personal safety around strangers.

Who Are Stranger Offenders?

Stranger offenders (hereafter called offenders) are people who abduct and/or abuse children they don't know. They do not seek a relationship with the child, as do abusers who know the child. Instead, they see children as objects for their use. They view children as weak, helpless, defenseless victims who can be manipulated easily to fulfill the offenders' needs.

These offenders range from the passive exhibitionist to the sadistic murderer. Bribery, flattery, treats, and requests for help are common tricks they use to engage children. **While some strangers will actually snatch a child away, this rarely happens.** Most children are lured into a seemingly innocent situation with someone who acts like a "nice" person.

Of particular concern are those pedophiles who "hang out" in places where they have access to children: fast food restaurants, arcades, malls, movies, mini-markets, etc. These offenders will engage a child, molest them in the bathroom or other readily available area, and then release the child. These perpetrators tend to prefer boys and report molesting hundreds of children in this manner.

Because there is no way to anticipate who these offenders are or what they will do, the best defense is to keep unsupervised children away from strangers. This is first and foremost the responsibility of parents and other responsible adults. But children also need to be educated, to learn rules that will reduce their risk when adult efforts to protect them fail.

Strangers—the Child's Point of View

Strangers have been the focus of so much of our concern for our children's safety that most children have a pretty distorted sense of who and what strangers are. What we've said about strangers makes sense to *us*, but doesn't usually make sense to them.

Children believe that the world is divided into two types of people: good guys and bad guys. We've traditionally taught them that the ones they need to worry about and watch out for are the bad guys. (Don't take candy from strangers; beware of strangers; stranger danger.) Of course, this is as impossible for children as it is for adults.

Teaching children to be afraid of strangers not only doesn't work very well, it is also frightening. When we say things like "Don't talk to strangers or get in their car because they might take

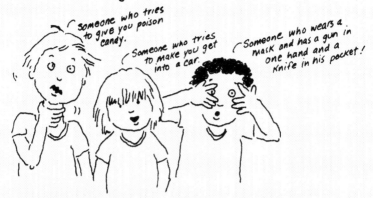

What is a stranger?

Someone who tries to give you poison candy.

Someone who tries to make you get into a car.

Someone who wears a mask and has a gun in one hand and a knife in his pocket!

you away and we'd never see you again," we scare children without protecting them.

Instead of using fear tactics, the Safe Child approach will teach you how to give your children specific guidelines and information to limit their vulnerability while maintaining their ability to move freely in their everyday lives.

What Bad Guys Look Like

Young children see strangers as people who want to hurt little kids, who will try to lead them into dangerous situations, and who can be recognized because they *look bad*. From a child's point of view, staying safe is simply a matter of watching out for bad people who look like their idea of a stereotypical stranger. Following that logic, everyone else is okay. And, yet, we know that isn't true.

I especially remember one child who said, "A stranger is someone who wears a Band-Aid on his head." When I questioned him, he explained that his mother had said strangers hurt children because "they're a little bit sick up here," pointing to his head. Most of what we've said to children about strangers is distorted and misunderstood.

Some children will say a stranger is "someone you don't know." But when you ask them what a stranger looks like, you get

Identifying Strangers

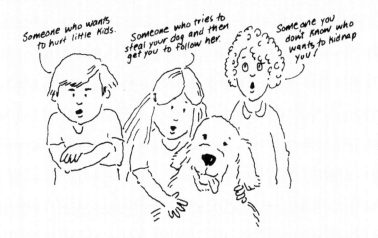

stereotypical answers, such as: "They're dirty, with messed-up hair." "They have long fingernails and torn shoes." Or "They're kind of sleazy-looking, with shifty eyes."

The real danger to our children lies in their belief that "good" guys are easily distinguished from "bad" guys by how they look. As adults, we know that strangers who are dangerous are often kind, solicitous, friendly, and normal-looking.

How Do You Tell?

If visual cues aren't the answer, then what do you say to your children? First, help them understand that there is no way to tell by the way someone looks how they are on the inside. With younger children, you might ask, "Could you misbehave when you were dressed up in your best clothes?" Conversely, "Are you bad on the inside because you're wearing a mean witch's costume on the outside?"

With older children, you should talk about stereotypes. They should know that judging someone by their appearance is a mistake.

Goodness and badness are not visible traits. Children who believe they can tell the good guys from the bad guys by how they look are in danger.

The Safe Child Book

A Stranger Is Anyone You Don't Know

Children need to learn about strangers: not any one type of stranger in particular, but strangers in general, so that they can apply the safety rules.

Tell your children that most strangers are good, kind, friendly people. In fact, every single one of their new sitters, teachers, coaches, doctors, etc., are strangers when they first meet them. Most of them turn out to be people your children like and trust.

The world is also full of people who want to be around children. Most of these people are genuinely nice. Some aren't. To illustrate this, talk to your children about a grouchy neighbor or someone who seemed nice at first but turned out not to be. The central message is: You can't tell nice people from not-very-nice people by how they look.

Preparing to Change the Rules

The rules I teach children regarding strangers build upon two simple ideas. **The first is that there is only one person who is with you all the time, who can be responsible for keeping you safe, all the time. That person is you.**

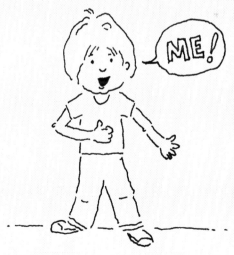

Identifying Strangers

Most children believe that grown-ups keep them safe all the time. Children do not realize, until they are well into first grade, that they are on their own much of the time. It is important that even young children understand that Mom, Dad, teacher, and even baby-sitter are not always there. They need to know that they are responsible for following the rules in order to keep themselves safe *when they are by themselves.*

When talking about this idea with very young children, it is easier for them to understand by asking questions like:

"Who's the only person in the room when you're in the bathroom all by yourself?"

"Who's the only person there when you're playing in the backyard and I go in to answer the telephone?"

"Who's the only person who is with you all the time?"

"Then, who's the only person who can take care of you and keep you safe when you're all by yourself?"

"That's right, you are. Mom and Dad and your teachers and friends and the police are here to help and to teach you. But when you're by yourself, you need to pay attention and keep yourself safe."

The second basic idea is that when children are alone, it is their job to take care of themselves. It is not their job to take care of the adults in the world. If an adult needs assistance, he or she must get it from another adult, not from a child.

One of the primary ways children get hurt with strangers is by being friendly and helpful. If they understand that taking care of themselves is their first priority when they're alone, they have permission to ignore or deny adult requests for assistance.

Establishing a Common Ground

Children don't see the problem of strangers and abduction in the same way that parents do. **Our goal is to have clear, concrete rules that prevent problem situations, that enable chil-**

dren to function safely, and that still allow them to perceive the world as a fundamentally safe and nurturing place.

While the four rules outlined in the next chapter often seem stringent to adults, children slot them in along with all the other rules in their lives, like brushing their teeth and making the bed. In teaching these rules to thousands of children, I've consistently found that children are glad to have clearly defined rules about strangers. They are more comfortable knowing what is expected of them in a wide range of situations. You'll also feel more secure knowing that your children know what to do.

8

Preventing Abuse and Abduction by Strangers

The rules children learn about strangers should be simple, straightforward, and practical. The rules in this chapter tell children *exactly* what to do in a wide variety of situations. They also provide guidelines for situations that are unpredictable. Keep in mind that they should be taught without fear or anxiety and without suggesting to your children that anyone wants to hurt them.

Rule Number 1: The Arm's Reach Plus Rule

The first way to maximize the safety of children *when they are not in the presence of a caretaking adult* is to keep them an Arm's Reach Plus away from people they don't know.

An Arm's Reach Plus is the length of an adult's arm plus the distance reached when the adult bends over, plus a little bit more. The reason children need to stay at this distance is *not* because the person might want to hurt them. Rather, when they're by themselves, they need to keep a circle of safety around themselves. Staying an arm's reach away keeps them out of reach. This gives them the measure of safety they need if they feel uncomfortable about any situation and want to get out of it. It is perfectly appropriate behavior. It also avoids the nonsense of children running away whenever they see or are spoken to by a person they don't know. Additionally, if the person is an offender, it signals him or her that this child is not an easy target.

Three- to Seven-Year-Olds

For children as young as three and as old as six or seven, the game begins by teaching your children what an Arm's Reach Plus is:

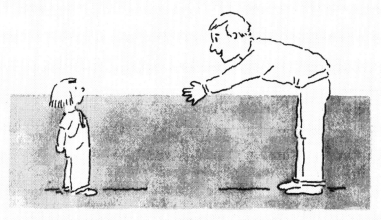

"If you were playing in the front yard and someone you didn't know—a stranger—came into the yard, I'd want you to stay an Arm's Reach Plus away from that person. They might be a friend of Mom or Dad that you don't know. They might be anybody. What I want you to do is pay attention and stay an Arm's Reach Plus away. Could you do that? Let's pretend. I'll be the stranger. . . ."

Once your children understand how far away you want them to be, you can begin to illustrate the rule's use by acting out "What If . . ." Do this by role-playing, by walking through the story and guiding your children as you go along. **Talking about this rule doesn't make sense to children. You need to show them what you mean and then practice.** This should be done in a relaxed manner, without fear. Remember to weave through the entire game the idea that the person you're pretending to be is probably a nice person, but you can't tell by appearances, so you have to follow the rules.

The process of teaching the Stand Up, Back Up, and Run To . . . game is illustrated below:

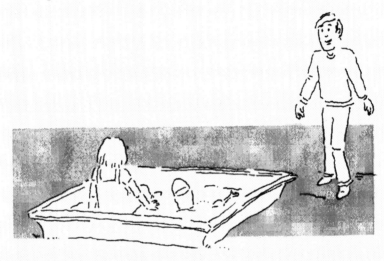

"Okay, now Dad will be the stranger. What if you were playing in the sandbox and a stranger came into the yard? You'd need to stand up as soon as you saw that it was someone you didn't know and then back up if the person came over to talk to you."

The Safe Child Book

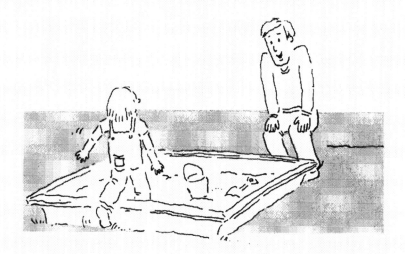

"The person might be very nice and start talking to you and might even know your name. What would you do?"

"That's right, you wouldn't talk to them, you'd just pay attention and stay an Arm's Reach Plus away. If the person took a step toward you, you should back up. If the person took another step, you'd back up again. Very good!"

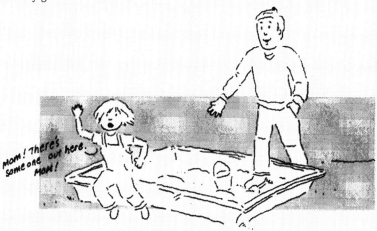

"If you get nervous or scared, I want you to back up four more steps and turn and run into the house as quickly as you can. I want you to yell really loudly so Mom or Dad will know you're coming and that you need us. Could you do that every single time you feel even a little bit scared? Good!"

Preventing Abuse and Abduction by Strangers

Seven Years Old and Older

The Arm's Reach Plus Rule is no less valuable for older children. They have more opportunities to be out with friends and are more vulnerable in some ways, especially to those offenders who are looking to molest a child in a public place such as a theater, arcade, or sports arena.

Having discussed the idea that there isn't any way to tell the good guys from the bad guys, you may introduce the Arm's Reach Plus Rule:

"Let's say you were someplace where there weren't a lot of people around, like a field or playground, and you saw someone walking toward you. Do you think it would be smart to stay far enough away from that person so that you could get out of there if you began to feel weird about what was happening?"

As children get older, fear of looking foolish or being embarrassed are major barriers. They are much more aware of "how things look" and often hesitate to follow their instincts because "What if . . ." the stranger turned out to be a "nice person."

It's worthwhile to share experiences you've had as an adult when you failed to do the right thing to keep yourself safe because you felt silly or embarrassed. For example, one question worth discussing with older children is, "Would it be embarrassing to stop what you're doing and back away if a stranger was approaching you? I think it might be, but sometimes we have to choose between being embarrassed and being safe."

Discuss how the Arm's Reach Plus Rule might apply if someone approaches them in a public place or if someone is uncomfortably close or paying too much attention to them in an arcade, a mall, or at a sports event. Would they be willing to walk away from a video game to get help or go to an area where their friends can be more available? Would they be willing to tell the person to leave them alone, or to make a scene that could draw attention to what was happening? How would that feel? How would they balance their feelings of ambivalence or embarrassment and their safety?

Rule Number 2: Don't Talk to Strangers

This rule is an old one. It seems obvious and yet, for most children, if I walked into the yard and said, "Hi, my name's Sherryll, what's yours?" they would immediately answer me. We teach our children to be polite. We often ask them to say hello to total strangers. **As a result, children think it is more important to be polite than to be safe.**

In order to change this, you must give your children specific permission not to respond to a friendly hello from a stranger. Keep in mind, this rule applies only when they are alone or with their friends, not when they are with an adult.

In fact, it is very helpful for your children to talk to strangers when you are present. It is an opportunity for you to teach appropriate behavior with adults and to deal with your children's expressions of comfort or discomfort with the various people they meet.

If your children are hesitant to talk to a stranger, even if that stranger is a good friend of yours, you should support them. Let your children know that you trust their instincts and personal preferences.

As children get older, you may gradually relax this rule to suit their maturity. For example, by age nine or ten, children may be comfortable saying hello in response to a casual hello on the street. That may be fine, but it is *not* okay for that hello to turn into a conversation, or a question-and-answer session.

Likewise, in an arcade, swimming pool, or other public area, children may be comfortable saying hello, but it is not all right to become engaged in a conversation unless a parent or other supervising adult is right there. It is also important to establish that this does not make the person a friend or acquaintance. If they see the person in the dressing room later (when a parent is not there), it is not safe to continue the discussion or to continue to be around the person. Again, you might discuss whether your child would be willing to make a scene, to attract attention when he becomes uncomfortable with what is happening.

By age nine or ten, children also may feel comfortable answering a request for directions from someone in a car, if and only if they are at least ten feet away from the car and they are able to answer the question simply. If the person asks them to look at an address, draw a map, or do anything requiring them to come closer, they need to end the exchange and go to an area with other people.

It is important to point out that just because children begin to help someone doesn't mean that they can't stop *at any point* if they feel uncomfortable. This may seem rude and, perhaps, irrational. Nevertheless, they need to trust their instinct and do whatever *they* feel they need to do for their own safety.

But They Knew My Name . . .

How many times have we seen children instantly perk up at the sound of their name? They are completely disarmed, thinking that you know them if you know their name. How often I have heard children say, "He wasn't a stranger, he knew my name and he told me his name."

Children are easily tricked into giving their names. One offender regularly started with "Hi, Larry," 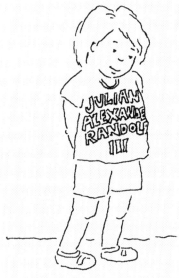 to which children responded, "I'm not Larry, I'm ———." He then started a conversation, and when the children later recalled what happened, they all thought he had known their names.

Talk to your children about some of the ways a stranger could know their names. This might include reading their name on a shirt, belt, book, or bicycle tag, or hearing a friend, teacher, or parent call the child by name. You can help solve this problem by avoiding the use of clothing, barrettes, lunch boxes, etc., with your children's names displayed on them. Label their clothing and other possessions where the name will not be visible. If you already have items of clothing marked with your children's names, save them for times when you are going to be with them.

Talk to your children's teachers about the use of name tags on field trips and the presence of parents, unfamiliar to the children, as trip helpers. One solution to this problem is the use of color or shape tags (bears, apples, birds) to be worn by children and leaders. Anyone without a proper tag would be immediately recognized as separate from the group and the children would know to find someone with a tag like their own.

This is equally true for older children. I will often call a fifth or sixth grader by name all the way through a class because he has his name on the back of his sports jersey. At the end of the class, I always ask if he knows how I knew his name. I cannot remember a time when the answer wasn't "Oh, I figured you knew my mom and dad or something." *Older children think they are at lower risk of abuse and abduction. So do their parents. This is, at least in part, what makes them so vulnerable.*

As simple as these rules seem, they are for all children. **If children hesitate to follow the rules because they were called by name, their level of safety decreases sharply. Knowing someone is more than exchanging names.**

Rule Number 3: Don't Take Things from Strangers—Not Even Your Own Things

While this rule also seems obvious, it is not. Children think that it means not taking things like candy, toys, or animals. To make this rule relevant, we need to use examples that are plausible and reflect everyday situations. We also need to be clear that this is a rule that applies *only* when children are not with a caretaking adult.

When children are with an adult and someone offers candy, samples, or other treats, they should be taught to

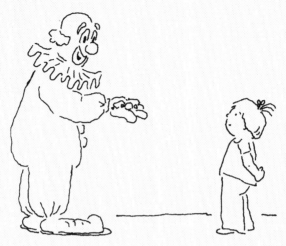

ask permission before taking it. When they are by themselves or with their friends, they must never take anything from someone they don't know.

Three- to Seven-Year-Olds

Begin with concrete stories and role-play.

For example: "What if someone you didn't know came up to you and said, 'Your dad left his keys at work and he wanted me to give them to you.' What would you do?" Act this out. Your child should stop what he or she is doing, stand up, back up, pay attention, not talk, and not take the keys.

This sounds complex. It is not. Preschoolers do it easily when you act this out rather than talk about it.

Young children can be fooled by a familiar make-believe character. They should know that even characters in costume are not an exception to the rule when they are by themselves.

I think my most poignant experience teaching this rule was when a five-year-old in one of my classes explained to me, "But what if someone said, 'Come here, little girl, and look at my bunnies.' I wouldn't, but what if they were just peeking up out of the box a little bit and all I could see were their little eyes and ears and paws, and they looked so cute. It would be really hard, wouldn't it?" Children understand that following the rules isn't always easy.

The Safe Child Book

One special "What If . . ." to play with your preschoolers portrays a stranger who walks into the yard, picks up one of your child's favorite toys, and tries to hand it to him or her. This is probably the most difficult "What If . . ." I do with children. They teeter back and forth because they want their toy, but they want to follow the rule.

When you play this "What If . . .," tell your child you know how hard it is, but that he or she is more important than the toy. One effective way to say this is: "If something happened to your doll, could we go to the store and buy a new one? Sure we could. If something happened to you, could we go to the store and buy another you? Of course not, that's silly. So as much as you love your doll, you're more important than she is. Mom and Dad love you more." Once children understand this, it is easier for them not to take a favorite toy from a stranger, but to come and tell you instead.

Eight Years and Older

As children get older, this rule is no less important. For example, "What if you were in the yard and a lady walked up with a book in her hand? She says she's a friend of your mom's and needs to get this book to her by tonight. Do you take it?" The answer is no, because children do not take things from people they don't know, not even to be helpful.

In using this role-play over the years, it has been insightful. Most preadolescent children tell me that the reason they don't take the book is it might have poison ink! The subject of strangers is distorted, even for older children.

Remind your children it is not their responsibility to take care of your book. The adult can leave it on the porch, put it in the mailbox, or make other arrangements. This may seem overly cautious, but most children who get hurt by strangers are drawn in by apparently reasonable and harmless requests. **We cannot ask our children to judge situations involving strangers by the rationality of the request any more than by the appearance of the stranger.**

An excellent "What If . . ." to explore the range of difficulties a situation can create would be: "What if your chain comes off your bicycle when you're at the park? You're working on it, trying to fix it. Someone approaches you and offers to help. When you back away, they steal your bike. What do you do? Would you be afraid to come home and tell us?"

Most of the "What If . . ."s I use come from actual incidents. In this case, a professional associate told me about the day his son came home with a black eye and many cuts and bruises. Someone had stolen his bicycle. When his father asked why he hadn't just let them have it, the son replied, "Because I knew you'd be mad if I didn't at least try to get it back."

Children should be very clear that you value them more than their possessions. While *you* know this, most children will sacrifice themselves for their toys, at least in part, because they're afraid they'll get in trouble if they come home without them.

Rule Number 4: Don't Go Anywhere with a Stranger

Most children know not to go anywhere with a stranger. That's why strangers make up such good stories.

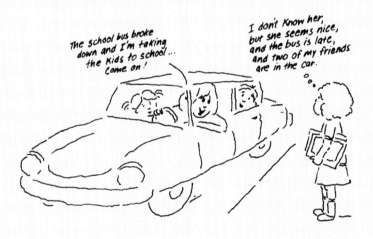

The school bus broke down and I'm taking the kids to school... Come on!

I don't know her, but she seems nice, and the bus is late, and two of my friends are in the car.

The Safe Child Book

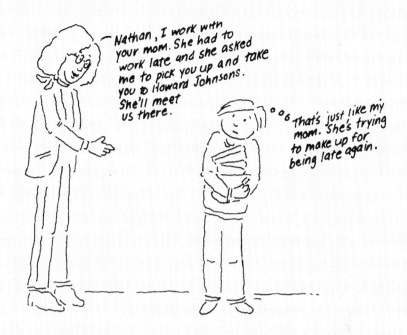

In both cases, the rule is clear. If Mom or Dad hasn't told you ahead of time that it's okay to go, you don't go.

Here are a few more examples:

"What if someone you didn't know came and said your dog had been hurt and you had to come right away?"

"What if a stranger showed up at the basketball game and said I'd had a flat tire and I asked him to take you to the gas station to meet me?"

"What if a neighbor, or someone else you know, came and said I'd told them to pick you up, but I hadn't said anything to you about it? Would you go?"

It is important that your children know what they can expect from you. Otherwise, they take too much time to consider what the stranger is saying. This is time during which they could be in extreme danger. They need to be able to recognize immediately that this is not part of the rules the family has agreed upon and that they should go for help.

The Code Word

The code word is an agreement that you make with your children, ages six or seven and up. It says, "If I ever send someone, other than who I said I would send, to pick you up, they will know the code word. If they don't know the code word, don't ever go with them, no matter what they tell you." The code word can be anything: a word or even a sentence.

Children love using the code word. The code word easily and safely puts your children in charge of the situation. Once a code word is used, children may want to change it. That's fine. There is no limit to the number of code words. Allow your children to use it and change it as they need to, as long as everyone always knows what the current code word is.

Parents are sometimes careless about messages. For example, when you call your child's school and leave a message that is passed along by the sixth-grade monitor to the teacher, and from the teacher to your child, a margin of safety is lost. Whenever possible, give your messages directly to your children. Permission via someone else is not valid permission except in certain clearly defined cases. Your children should always get permission from the source—you.

For children who may be at higher risk for abduction (as in some custody cases), a code word can be used with the school. The child would never be released except to someone having the code word. I strongly recommend that you test this system before relying on it, as some schools are lax about enforcement of such an agreement.

Feeling Funny Inside

Above and beyond all the rules, especially for older children, instinct, "that funny feeling inside," is their most important friend. Once children are in a dangerous or

compromised situation, instinct must guide their decisions about how to survive.

For children's purposes, instinct is most simply defined this way: **Instinct is nature's way of talking to you and helping to keep you safe.**

Children talk about instinct in many ways and it is difficult to define, even for adults. Whatever description children give for where or how they feel their own instincts is fine. What's important is that they recognize it so they'll know how to "listen" to it.

"What If They Get Me Anyway?"

At some point, children may ask, "What if they get me anyway?" This possibility *should not* be brought up until children ask. At that point, talk about your children's feelings. Help them to understand that it is impossible to create a rule for what they should do in every situation. Only their understanding of what is happening and their assessment of what they should do can guide them during a specific incident.

The best choice is usually to do anything they possibly can to attract attention while they are still in a public place. They can kick and scream and do anything else in their power to get away. On the other hand, if they are abducted and their instinct tells them to be quiet and compliant and look for a chance to sneak away or wait to be let go, that is what they should do.

Talk about how they might get in touch with you. Be certain your children know where they live, their full address and phone number, and how to make a local or long-distance call, even if they have no money. Be sure they know you would always want to know where they were, no matter what someone said to the contrary.

I want to stress that this is a subject for discussion only when your children bring it up. Your job is to give them information that addresses their concerns to teach the applicable rules and strategies using nonfearful examples.

Children Prevent Abuse and Abduction

As with sexual abuse by people known to the child, there are limits to the precautions parents can take to protect their children from abuse and abduction by strangers. Strangers approach children when they are alone or with a group of friends. For that reason, your children must be prepared to take care of themselves when they're not with you.

Children also can be active in protecting siblings, friends, and other children. Discuss what appropriate actions they might take if they see a child acting unsafely. Emphasize the importance of telling an adult right away.

If your children go places with minimal supervision, put all the rules together. Use scenarios that call upon all the rules. For example, in an arcade where there are many people mingling, it is not all right to become engaged in a conversation, to take money, or go to another area of the facility with someone they don't know, no matter what they look or act like or what the person has to offer. This is a good example of what the rules mean in everyday life.

Be confident in your responsibility to limit your children's activities until you are sure they can handle the freedom of movement you give them. The decisions you make for your children should be based on what you know about their ability to follow the rules and your assessment of their maturity.

You don't do it alone. Protecting children from abuse and abduction by strangers is a partnership between you and your children. If you teach your children about strangers as positively and clearly as you teach them to cross the street, they will not only have a healthier attitude about the world, they will be safer.

The Stranger Rules Checklist

- A stranger is anyone you don't know.

- You can't tell the good guys from the bad guys by how they look.

- You are responsible for keeping yourself safe when you're by yourself.

- You are responsible only for taking care of yourself; you are not responsible for grown-ups. Adults who need help should go to another adult.

- Instinct is nature's way of talking to you—listen to that inner voice.

The four stranger rules you should always follow when you're not with an adult who is taking care of you are:

1. Stay an Arm's Reach Plus away from strangers. Stand up, back up, and run to someone who can help you if you feel afraid.

2. Don't talk to strangers.

3. Don't take anything from strangers—not even your own things.

4. Don't go anywhere with a stranger.

9

Staying Alone

Current estimates of the number of children left in self-care range from 7 percent to 25 percent of the nation's 30 million school-age children. These large differences in estimates exist partly because of inconsistent definitions of self-care and because parents are reluctant to give out this information. Guilt, social stigma, and awareness that leaving their children unattended may appear irresponsible or be considered neglectful have prevented many parents from reporting their child-care methods accurately.

Even if you think you *never* leave your children alone, realistically, you need to deal with the issues: you're in the shower and someone comes to the door; or you're in the garden and the phone rings. With only the rarest exceptions, all children are alone at one time or another. You probably wonder, and I know children wonder, about what could happen at those times. Knowing what to do in a variety of circumstances not only reassures children, but it also prepares them to be safer.

In a nationwide research effort I led in 1988, we developed a new method for assessing incidence of self-care. In a sample of 447 families with children in kindergarten through grade three in rural, urban, and suburban settings, we found the following:

- Thirty-five percent of these children were left in self-care occasionally.

- Seven percent of these children were left in self-care regularly.

Perhaps more important, we learned about the attitudes and behaviors of these parents. Urban children were far more often left unattended. These parents tended to be matter-of-fact about their child-care decisions. They consistently noted resources that they had arranged for their children, such as a neighbor or relative available in the apartment building or neighborhood.

Suburban parents were less likely to leave their children in self-care on a regular basis but were considerably more likely to leave them unattended for the "occasional" trip to the store. These parents did not generally perceive themselves as leaving their children alone and were much less likely to have discussed safety issues with their children.

Rural parents cited the isolation of the rural setting and the inability of younger children to get to a neighbor quickly as a reason for not leaving their children alone on a regular basis. However, they were as likely as suburban parents to leave their children alone for the occasional errand.

In addition to looking at incidence of self-care, we created an opportunity for parents to learn how well their children were doing at following the guidelines they had set. With sixteen of the children who were regularly left in self-care, we placed a phone call to the child and then a few minutes later attempted to deliver a package to the house. The results were startling in terms of what they told these families about actual risk to their children.

Only two of the sixteen children handled the telephone call properly. All of the other children readily spoke with the evaluator, offering information that included their name and the fact that they were home alone.

None of the children handled the package delivery appropriately. Thirteen of the children opened the door and took the package. Two children pretended not to be at home (increasing the risk to the child if a perpetrator believes no one is at home).

The last child was playing in the street and happily told us no one was at home and he would take the package. In the debriefing interviews with parents, all expressed surprise at their children's actions. Each parent believed his or her child would have refused to open the door.

Although this is a small number of children, the findings are compellingly clear. At the very least, these children are at risk, vulnerable to people from the outside. Additionally, if they aren't prepared to handle these everyday events safely, it must be anticipated that they are unprepared to handle other problems, including emergencies.

Finally, the striking difference between the expectations of parents and the actual performance of their children tells us that parents are not realistically assessing their children's ability to handle even the most common occurrences. The purpose of this chapter is to help you to make your child-care choices and to provide your children with maximum skills to insure their own safety when they are without supervision.

Leaving children to care for themselves is a controversial issue. I will not make a case for or against it. If you are going to leave your children alone, you need to make them as safe as possible. Talk with your children about the feelings and concerns they have when they're alone, even if only for a few minutes. Discuss the various issues in this chapter so they know what you expect of them. Give them a sense of control, if not choice, in the decisions being made about their care, particularly if they are left alone on a regular basis.

Ground Rules for Self-Care

If your children are left alone before or after school or when you go out, clear ground rules are essential. The "What If . . ." game is a natural way to go over the wide range of things that come up when your children are by themselves. They should know when to be home, how far from home they can go, whether they can have friends in, what snacks they can have, when to do their homework, what TV they can watch, etc.

The following checklist can be used to make sure your children know their name, address, and phone number. Use it also to give them emergency numbers, to establish basic rules, and to set expectations.

STAYING ALONE CHECKLIST

My name:	**Neighbors:**
My parents' names:	**Police:**
My address:	**Fire:**
My phone number:	**Doctor:**
Resource people:	**Work:**

Other

If the phone rings, I will:	**If someone comes to the door, I will:**
If there is an emergency:	**If I get bored:**
If I get scared:	**My responsibilities are:**

Negotiating Ground Rules

One of the greatest concerns for parents who leave their children alone is deciding what limits to set. Children are pressing for more freedom while parents are trying to hold the line for the sake of safety and structure. Negotiating limits furnishes an important opportunity to discuss safety and personal responsibility.

I use a simple chart to list the privilege desired on one side and the associated responsibilities on the other. Children are amazingly good at coming up with the responsibilities associated with a privilege. They can often articulate your concerns better than you can.

For example, children often want to be able to have friends in when they stay alone. In this situation, and many others as children get older, the following privileges and responsibilities exercise will help you look carefully at the privileges your children want, the responsibilities that go with them, and to agree on the limits.

PRIVILEGE	RESPONSIBILITIES
1. I want to be able to have a friend over after school, even if there's no adult here.	1. We won't talk on the phone too long. 2. We won't go outside the yard. 3. We'll watch my little brother. 4. We'll do our homework.

Once the chart is complete, discuss it. If your children feel they are up to the responsibilities, you may grant them the privilege for a test period. *The beauty of this approach is that children will sometimes look at the list and decide they don't want, or can't handle, the privilege just yet.* Another benefit is that if children are unable to meet the responsibilities, the privilege is withdrawn, and the children—not you—are responsible for the loss of the privilege.

One of my favorite applications of this exercise is with preadolescent girls who want a horse. After detailing all the responsibilities that go with a horse, including the expenses, they are able to see that they may want a horse but it is impossible for them to assume the responsibilities and expenses.

Answering the Telephone

Parents often think their children know how to use the telephone when they don't. Have your children show you that they can use the telephone. If you have an autodialer you may want to put pictures of people next to the numbers so your young children can call quickly and easily in an emergency. For older children, they should understand how telephones work. This seems obvious, but with the new technologies, I've encountered more than one phone that I couldn't figure out.

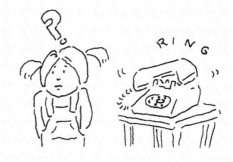

Answering Machines and Voice Mail

Answering machines and voice mail have complicated parental decisions about children answering the telephone when they're home alone. Reasons for having them answer the telephone include:

- It is your line of communication with them.

- It can be frightening for children to sit and listen to the phone ring and ring, not knowing who it might be.

- Burglars often call first to find out if anyone's home.

On the other hand, it is increasingly common for people to screen calls with an answering machine. If you choose to do this, be sure your children know how to pick up without erasing all your messages. Be clear about when they should pick up the phone and when they should let the machine take the message.

Voice mail does not provide these options and has the disadvantages listed earlier. If you choose to use voice mail, be sure you have a signal that enables you to get in touch with your children, such as: ring two times, hang up, and call back.

Safe Telephone Procedures for General Calls

When your children do answer the telephone, the following guidelines should be considered:

- Answer the phone with "Hello," not with a first or last name, such as "This is Lisa" or "Williams residence." Children should not give their name out or answer any questions over the phone unless they are talking to a family member or close family friend.

- When children are home alone, they should say, "My mom is busy, may I take a message?" or "My dad is lying down, may I take a message?"

- If needed, your child should take the message. (I strongly recommend carbon message pads and an attached pencil beside every telephone to emphasize that message-taking is a serious responsibility and to provide a backup for lost messages.)

- If the caller doesn't wish to leave a message, children should say good-bye and hang up the phone.

- If your children cannot take messages, for whatever reason, they should ask the caller to call back.

Special Calls

Prank calls. Whether they are silly ("Have you got Prince Albert in a can?") or threatening ("I'm following you"), children should hang up immediately. Prank callers need a response in order to "play their game." When they don't get it, they usually stop.

Repeated prank calls. Whether they are made by children or adults, whether they are silly or threatening, if someone keeps calling and calling, especially if it's frightening, children should call a parent or another adult for help.

Sales calls. Interrupt and say "No, thank you," then hang up the phone. It is not rude for children to interrupt if the person keeps talking.

Survey calls. Say "No, thank you" and hang up the phone, even if the caller offers a free prize or money to children in exchange for answering the questions.

Question calls. Do not answer anyone's questions over the phone. Say "No, thank you" and hang up. Even if the caller says your child must answer the questions, it is not true. Children should know that no one has to answer questions over the phone. It is all right to hang up.

"I'm watching you" calls. This is usually a trick or a prank call by someone the children know. If you think about it, most children come home from school, go to the kitchen to make a snack, and turn on the television. So someone who calls and says, "I can see you. You're in the kitchen making a snack. Now do everything I say," is making a pretty safe guess about any child after school. As with any other prank call, the thing to do is hang up. If children feel frightened in this or any other situation, they should call someone for help.

The key to safety with all telephone calls is: *your children are in control.* Hanging up is always an acceptable way to handle a problem caller.

Answering the Door

Children should *always* go to the door and ask who is there, but *not open* it, when they are home alone. **Children who pretend they're not home feel frightened and powerless. They are also in danger be-**

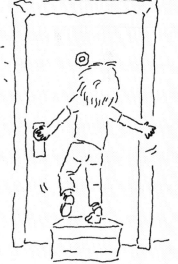

cause burglars usually knock first and prefer not to enter an occupied home. Remember: Children *should not open the door for anyone* except a member of the family or a friend if they have permission.

When children are home alone, they are responsible for themselves. They do not need to be helpful to someone who comes to the door. It is important that your children are comfortable saying no, even to someone with a good story.

Safe Door Procedures

Children who are home alone should:

* Always keep the house locked.

* Always go to the door.

* Say "Who is it?"

* Not open the door for anyone except a member of the family or a friend, if they have permission.

* Say "My mother is in the shower" or "My father is on the telephone" if the person asks for their parents.

* Have the package left outside if the person has a delivery.

* Send the person to a neighbor or have him come back later if the delivery requires a signature.

* Not open the door if there has been an accident or an emergency and someone wants to use the phone. They can call 911 and ask for help.

* Not allow anyone other than designated family and friends into the house for any reason. Children should not agree to open the door "just a little bit" to anyone they don't know.

Being Scared: Fear Versus Being Spooked

There is a significant difference between being frightened and feeling increasingly anxious when you're home alone. Ask your children what frightens them. Talk about how it feels to be spooked versus how it feels to be afraid. Decide with them who it would be okay to call when they're just nervous about hearing noises and who they should call when it's a real emergency.

Knowing Normal Noises

This is an enjoyable and easy exercise that identifies the noises that are always around but that we don't hear until we begin feeling scared. To do this exercise, sit down with your children and listen very carefully to the noises in and outside the house. Write down all the noises you hear: the refrigerator motor, the heating system, a branch scraping on the window, snow shifting on the roof, whatever. This exercise should be repeated from time to time because household noises change at different times of the year, and even different times of the day. When children know what the normal noises are, they won't get spooked so easily.

Emergencies

Although we pay lip service to emergency preparedness, most families don't even have an emergency escape route for fires. Most parents don't discuss how to get out of the house if a burglar should enter. Most families don't have basic first aid supplies or training. **Since the three most common emergency situations are fires, robberies, and accidents, this lack of preparation creates a life-threatening situation for children, especially those who stay alone regularly.**

I've had many revealing conversations with children about how they handle basic emergencies. Following are some common responses to "What if . . ." questions:

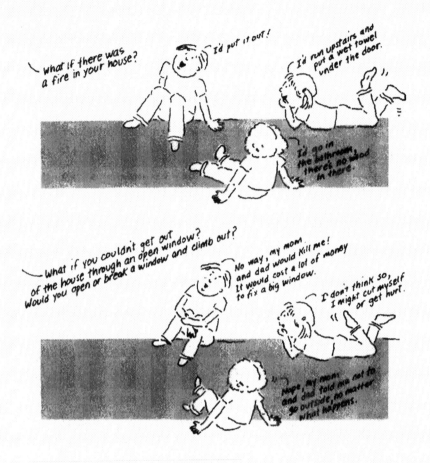

This is only one of the frightening examples of how literally our children take what we say to them. It points out the need to structure personal safety training so children learn to think about the situations they're in rather than blindly following the rules that apply to "safe" situations.

Children need to know what to do in an emergency, whom to call, and how to make an emergency call. They need to know that all the rules can change in a life-threatening situation and that they have your permission to do whatever needs to be done to protect themselves and each other.

Resources for Help

The single greatest feature cited by children who feel good about staying alone is the availability of their parents and other resource people. Knowing this, parents and employers should work together to make it easy for children to check in. It establishes a link so children can let someone know they're all right. It also means they know they have someone to call if they're not.

Having the option to call makes a difference in how children feel about being alone. If it's not possible for children to call Mom or Dad, designate someone else who can take that call, someone who will take a few minutes to chat, someone your children will feel comfortable talking to about a problem.

Staying Alone Safely

Leaving your school-age children by themselves, even for short periods of time, is a very personal choice. It can be a nurturing, satisfying, and safe experience if it is appropriately planned, discussed, and monitored. **Children who have siblings staying with them, neighbors who are willing to be a resource, and predetermined guidelines about chores, homework, television, recreation, etc., do better than children who are genuinely "on their own."**

If you leave your children alone, don't feel guilty. Staying alone can be a very positive learning opportunity for many children. Put your energy into making it safe and satisfying, both physically and emotionally. Prevention and ongoing discussions are the bywords.

10

Dealing with Bullies

Bullying is something most children encounter in one form or another. Children struggle with being called names, being picked upon, being excluded, not knowing how to make friends, or being the ones acting unkindly or aggressively toward others. All forms of bullying are abusive and all are opportunities to teach children how to get along, how to be considerate people, how to be part of a community or group.

Try to recall an experience you had when you were bullied, excluded, treated unkindly. The pain is intense. Fear, powerlessness, helplessness are the core feelings and responses to bullying. For many children, this dominates their school or neighborhood experience. For some, it is what they live with at home.

The United States Department of Justice and the National Association of School Psychologists estimate that 160,000 children miss school each day because of fear. They are afraid of being bullied, humiliated, and injured. They're not sure who's in charge or who will protect them. It is this pattern of fear and uncertainty that is, in part, responsible for the increasing number of children who carry weapons to school.

This chapter will give you an overview of the problem and some specific suggestions for intervening in bullying situations and for teaching your children what to do and how to get help with bullying.

Who Are the Bullies?

Bullying can take many forms: physical, emotional, verbal, or a combination of these. It may involve one child bullying another, a group of children against a single child, or groups against other groups (gangs). It is not unlike other forms of victimization and abuse in that it involves:

- an imbalance of power,

- differing emotional tones—the victim will be upset whereas the bully is cool and in control,

- blaming the victim for what has happened,

- lack of concern on the part of the bully for the feelings and concerns of the victim, a lack of compassion.

Bullies are very often children who have been bullied or abused themselves. Sometimes, they are children experiencing life situations they can't cope with, that leave them feeling helpless and out of control. They may be children with poor social skills, who do not fit in, who can't meet the expectations of their family or school. They bully to feel competent, successful, to control someone else, to get some relief from their own feelings of powerlessness.

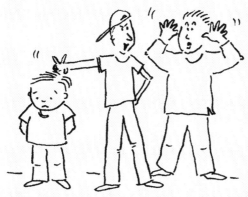

Who Are the Victims?

Not all children are equally likely to be victimized by bullying behavior. Those children who are more prone to be picked upon tend to have the following characteristics:

- Low self-esteem

- Insecurity

- Lack of social skills, don't pick up on social cues

- Cry or become emotionally distraught easily

- Unable to defend or stand up for themselves

Some children actually seem to provoke their own victimization. These children will tease bullies, making themselves a target by egging the person on, not knowing when to stop, and then not being able to defend themselves effectively when the balance of power shifts to the bully.

Children who are not bullied tend to have better social skills and conflict management skills. They are more willing to assert themselves about differences without being aggressive or confronting. They suggest compromises and alternate solutions. They tend to be more aware of people's feelings and are the children who can be most helpful in resolving disputes and assisting other children to get help.

If Your Child Is Being Bullied

Most children don't report that they are being bullied. Usually, parents learn about the bullying when they witness it, when another parent or child reports it, or when the school notifies the parent of a problem.

If you learn your child is being bullied, you may immediately want to protect your child and confront the aggressor. You may feel embarrassed and want your child to toughen up, to get in there and fight back. You may feel helpless yourself. None of these responses is helpful.

Get as much information as you can about what has happened. Avoid blaming anyone, including the bullying child or children. Look at your own child's behavior and style of interacting. Ask yourself what you know about your child and how you can turn the immediate situation around. Follow the suggestions in this chapter to further build your child's personal and interpersonal skills to reduce the likelihood of future victimization.

If you are going to get in touch with the parents of a bullying child, remember that they will probably feel defensive. Keep in mind that your goal is to have a safe and nurturing environment for all of the children, not to escalate an already difficult situation. In calling another parent, you might begin as follows:

1. "I'm Sy's mother. The kids aren't getting along and I wanted to tell you what I know about the problem and get your input on what we should do next." (This avoids name-calling and blaming.)

2. Describe what you know fully.

3. Ask what the other parent knows about the incident.

4. Request that the other parent work with his child (as you have with yours) to let the child know that aggression is not a way to solve problems, to talk about the feelings of both children, and to suggest alternative ways to handle the situation next time.

5. Invite the other parents to call you back if they have other ideas or would like to discuss the situation further after talking with their child.

6. Thank the other parents for taking the problem seriously and being responsive.

Dealing with Bullies

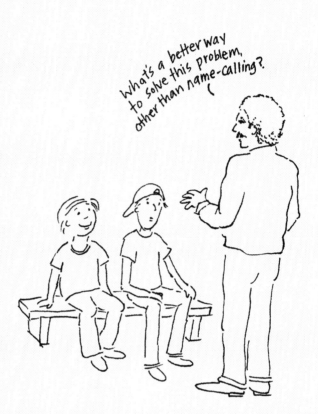

What's a better way to solve this problem, other than name-calling?

For your own children, there are several additional steps you can take.

1. Discuss alternatives to responding to bullies.

For example:

Don't react, walk away, get help if pursued. Agree with the bully, saying, "You're right," and walking away.

Be assertive. Remember tone of voice, body posture, words should be clear and assertive, not aggressive. "I don't want to be around anyone who talks that way" or "Leave me alone."

2. Role-play. Just as in prevention of child abuse, role-play is what makes the skills real. Actually walk through situations and have your child practice different responses.

3. Discuss prevention techniques.

For example:

Stay with other kids.

Do not get involved with bullies in any kind of interchange.

Don't take it personally, it's really the bullies' problems that are causing the situation, not you.

Invite the offending child over to play. Maybe she's struggling to find a way to be part of the group. Provide lots of activities and supervision to ensure that the play date is a positive one.

If Your Child Is the Bully

What every parent doesn't want to hear: your child is behaving like a bully. Your first response probably will be defensive. You may blame someone else's child, deny the accusation, say your child was provoked or misunderstood. You may feel angry and want to confront and punish your child. These are natural responses that aren't very helpful.

Disarm the situation and buy yourself some time to process what's being said. For example, "Instead of labeling my child, please tell me what happened." Make yourself really listen. Remember that this discussion is ultimately about the well-being of your child, regardless of how it's being framed. You need to know what's going on so you can take the most effective action to assist your child in learning to get along.

Even if your child is behaving aggressively or acting like a bully, remember that this behavior is probably coming from your child's feelings of vulnerability. You need to look for what is going on in your child's interactions with others and what is going on internally, causing your child to behave that way.

Keep in mind that the person who has told you about this is equally concerned about his/her own child and probably anxious about talking with you at all.

I suggest the following approach to this situation:

1. "Thank you for calling. I know it was probably hard to make this call."

2. "Bullying behavior is not acceptable. Please tell me everything you know about what happened."

3. "This is not acceptable behavior in our family. Let me talk with my child and I will get back to you."

In talking with your child, DO NOT BLAME. Do not get into a discussion about the whys of what happened. Your discussion should focus on several key points:

1. Bullying is not acceptable in our family or in society.

2. Here are some better ways to handle these types of situations.

3. If you are feeling frustrated or angry or aggressive, here are some things you can do. (Remember to role-play, act out the new behaviors.)

4. Develop your resources. Whom could you go to in school if you see yourself getting into this type of situation again? Who else could be helpful?

5. Specify concretely the consequences if the aggression or bullying continues. You want to stop the behavior, understand your child's feelings, then teach and reward more appropriate behavior.

Preventing Bullying

As soon as children begin to interact with others, we can begin to teach them not to be bullies and not to be bullied. We can give them words for their feelings, limit and change their behavior, and teach them better ways to express their feelings and wishes. Children do not learn to solve these kinds of problems and get along by themselves. We need to teach them.

For example, a two-year-old may grab a toy from another child. The other child may cry or grab it back or hit. This is your opportunity to intervene. Take the toy and say, "I know you want a turn with this toy, but it is not all right to grab it away and [to the other child] it is not all right to hit. You need to ask your friend to

The Safe Child Book

let you play with the toy or wait until he puts it down. If you need help, you can ask me." This acknowledges the feelings that are the source of the conflict, sets clear limits on unacceptable behavior, and offers a better approach.

When preschoolers begin to call people names or use unkind descriptions, intervene repeatedly and consistently. For example, your child points and says, "That kid's short and fat." Respond with: "Each of us is different. It would hurt his feelings to hear you say that and that's not all right."

In kindergarten, children learn the power of exclusion. We begin to hear things like: "She's not my friend and she can't come to my party." Respond with: "You don't have to be friends with her today, but it's not all right to make her feel bad by telling her she can't come to your party."

In the early elementary grades, cliques and little groups develop that can be quite exclusionary and cruel. Children need to hear clearly from us: "It's not all right to treat other people this way. How do you think she feels being told she can't play with you? How would it make you feel? How could you be a more thoughtful and kind person in this situation?" Kids don't have to play with everyone or even like everyone, but they can't be cruel about excluding others.

When new children move to the school or neighborhood, they may be victimized because they are new or different or withdrawn. The message from parents and teachers needs to be: "How could we make this child feel more welcome in the neighborhood? What could you do to introduce him to the other kids, to show him around the school, to make him feel more welcome?"

Boys who are physically small or weak are more prone to victimization. Making fun, picking on, and other forms of bullying should be identified in their earliest stages. The message needs to be crystal clear: "This is not okay. Think about how he must feel. How could you include him and let other kids know it's not all right to treat others this way?"

Children who are not bullies or victims have a powerful role to play in shaping the behavior of other children. Teach your children to speak up on behalf of children being bullied. "Don't treat her that way, it's not nice." "Hitting is not a good way to solve problems. Let's find a teacher and talk about what happened."

Teachers, Administrators, and Playground Aides

The greatest problem I have encountered in assisting children to learn good interpersonal and problem-solving skills is parents, teachers, administrators, and playground aides who say, "Let them work it out, they've got to learn to solve these kinds of problems on their own." NONSENSE!

Children do not learn to get along by fighting, by being unhappy, and feeling victimized. Hitting back does not stop bullying. It is the job of parents and schools to intervene and to use each of these altercations or instances of bullying as a teaching opportunity.

The process of learning to cooperate, to solve interpersonal conflicts, to stand up effectively for yourself and others, to respect individual differences and the feelings of yourself and others is not automatic. Children learn all of these essential interpersonal skills when we give them the words, when we show them how to get along, when we talk about their feelings and the feelings of others. This is the job of adults.

Safety on the Internet

Children tend to be way ahead of parents in cyberspace. For the most part, they are more comfortable with computer technologies, schools are going on-line rapidly, and the world is shrinking in totally new ways. Safety in this environment is an evolving issue, one that has attracted widespread media attention. The reality, however, of this technology is that it holds vastly more information, opportunity, and richness of experience than danger.

Parents need to understand the nature of this system. This chapter will give you a crash course on what the Internet is, how it works, how children access it, the inherent risks, safety suggestions, ground rules, and ways to monitor your children's participation in the Internet.

The Internet

The Internet physically is a computer network that literally links you via a telephone, computer, and modem with anyone else in the world. It is a global network of networks, thus the name "Internet."

The Internet began as a research project of the Department of Defense in the 1970s. In the 1980s, NASA and the National Science Foundation began to develop Internet systems that would allow scientists and computer centers around the world to exchange information and communicate directly and immediately. In the late 1980s, with the increase of low-cost computers and the explosion of computers into the home market, the number connected to the Internet also exploded. From only 200 connected computers in 1981, there were over 300,000 connected computers in 1991. In 1994, the number exceeded 3 million and today some estimates are that 50 million participants use the Internet.

The Internet is a social network. It connects you with the entire world. Communication is immediate and conversations can take place as easily and directly as with the telephone, only they occur in words, graphics, audio, and video.

The Internet is the most dramatic and dynamic library in the world and it comes directly to you. It is a way to get virtually any type of information. Through the Internet, you can access museums, libraries, government, interest groups, organizations, and this author. A few examples:

- Practice a language by finding a foreign pen pal or signing on with a language site.

- Play chess with someone anywhere in the world or just be a spectator.

- Browse recipes from all over the world, print what you want and cook.

- Get a look at resorts and vacation spots before you go.

- Visit a museum in another part of the world.

This is a resource that you must experience. It's like the prevention techniques I've discussed for your children. They are just concepts, an idea, until you practice them. The Internet is the same.

No question it is daunting, unknown, and intimidating—in your mind. In reality, it takes only about two hours to get comfortable using the Internet. The programs are self-guiding and what you can access is so fascinating that it doesn't really matter if you go someplace you didn't mean to go. Experiencing the Internet is the only way to understand its draw for children and adults alike, to support its profound value as a social and educational tool, and to be sufficiently informed to set ground rules and monitoring guidelines that will protect your children and your phone bill. Go to your library, college, or school and get on-line.

How It Works

The Internet generally is accessed through one of the on-line services, such as CompuServe, America On-line, AT&T, and Microsoft Network. There are also hundreds of independent services. There are several parts to the Internet that you should recognize.

E-mail is the private correspondence area of the Internet. It is a communication that goes from one party directly to another via the Internet. It is a part of the Internet where confidentiality is protected under the Electronic Communications Privacy Act.

Chat lines are open conversations that take place in various locations on the Internet. They can be joined by anyone and generally revolve around an area of interest. You can access a chat line and read all the past correspondence or just jump in and respond to the current discussion.

For example, to locate a pen pal from another part of the world, you can use the pen pals' news group section of the Internet to connect with a pen pal. Once a connection is made, the conversation can stay in the public chat line or move to private E-mail correspondence. This is one of the areas in which safety considerations come into play and will be discussed further below.

E-zines are electronic magazines. They allow users to scan information and when they hit an area of interest to access more information about it immediately. This is a good example of how hours and hours and lots of money can disappear on the Internet. It is like having all the museums, libraries, coffeehouses, interest groups, and your best friends available to you every time you go on-line.

The World Wide Web (WWW), or the Web, is the fastest-growing area of the Internet. The Web is a network within the Internet. A site or page on the Web is a location in which information is made available. For example, *The Safe Child Book* has a page on the Web (http://www.safechild.org). On that page, you can get updates from me on child safety issues, reviews of new books on child safety, information on school programs, and other tips.

Kids on the Internet

Common advice to parents suggests not allowing your kids to spend hours on the Internet. I don't automatically agree. If your child sat down with the encyclopedia and kept switching to different books to get deeper and deeper into an area of interest, you wouldn't object. This is child-driven learning. It is one of the best kinds of learning. It generates excitement and energy and a feeling of power. The fact that it occurs on the computer, rather than in a big, heavy set of books with very small print and no moving pictures, does not diminish its value.

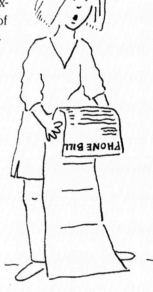

So the key issue is not the hours, it is a combination of the quality of the exchange occurring on the computer and balancing that with the other elements of life, such as physical activity, socialization, family, meeting responsibilities like homework, and getting a good night's sleep.

It is also a financial consideration. On-line time costs money in several ways. A service provider such as CompuServe charges an hourly fee. You may have to pay for a toll call if your provider is outside your local calling area. There is a fee for some programs that can be downloaded from the Internet. It's easy to run up usage bills of several hundred dollars every month. The telephone company and the on-line services don't care how the bill got there. It's yours to pay. Unless you're made of money, you must keep track of what your children are doing on the Internet. Obviously, then, it is important that children know how to get off-line as well as on-line.

In response to parental financial concerns, most on-line service providers now offer several important options that you should exercise:

- Contact the billing department and put a "cap" on your bill each month. You may do this by user or for the entire account. I recommend this even for yourself. This prevents an emergency interruption in which the system is left on-line, sometimes for days, without your knowledge.

- Look for an alarm clock in your options. Set it so there is an automatic reminder of time going by every thirty minutes.

- Keep a log of how much time is spent daily on-line. Teach your child to use the function that tells how long they were on-line.

- Use the internal log in your system. This will allow you to see what areas your children are using: E-mail, chat rooms, WWW.

Risks Using the Internet

There are two different safety issues on the Internet. The first is what your children are exposed to, either through their own ac-

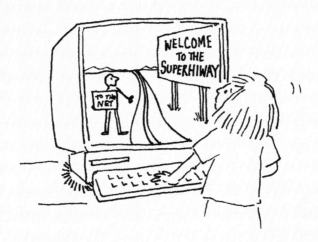

tions (entering an area that you may not want them to enter) or through accidental exposure.

The other distinct area of concern is direct communication with your child that may be inappropriate and personal and that could, if mishandled, lead to information being revealed that puts your child or the family at personal risk.

One of the things that people often find appealing about communication via the Internet is the element of anonymity. Children are able to communicate with anyone on the Net based on what and how they communicate. They are not limited by appearance, age, or other potentially prejudicial attributes. This is incredibly freeing. It's not uncommon for an adult to have a highly sophisticated conversation with someone on the Internet, believing the person to be an adult, only to find that he has been communicating with a teenager.

Conversations often become much more personal and intimate than they might in person because this element of anonymity frees some people to speak more openly and honestly. Extraordinarily close relationships can develop exclusively from Internet conversations. A feeling of trust can be cemented. STOP.

The unsettling reality is that all this can and does occur with a total stranger. All of what has been communicated may be true

The Safe Child Book

and none of it may be true. It is at the moment of trust, of deciding to make the next move, that the greatest areas of risk occur. Children and adults both have to STOP and look at what is really known, recognize the risks inherent in any decision to provide more personal information or to make a direct connection via E-mail, telephone, or in person. Adults are free to make those decisions. Children are not, and they should not be permitted to make these decisions.

Safety on the Internet

There are several ways to protect your children from exposure to pornography, explicit language, and other inappropriate interactions on the Internet. Use an on-line service that gives you good parental control. Familiarize yourself with your parental control center and use it to block:

1. *Chat rooms, forums, conference rooms, member rooms.* These are the areas of greatest risk for exposure to unwanted exchanges. They are not set up for children and are not a good way to spend their time or your money.

2. *Instant messages.* These are immediate person-to-person conversations that can only be viewed by the sender and receiver.

3. *Bulletin board services.* These again are freewheeling interest-driven exchange areas. They are not necessary for children.

4. *News groups.* You have the option to block all news groups or to use a program that blocks news groups by specific words. Programs are now available that help parents keep open access to appropriate news groups and to block all news groups with potentially explicit material.

5. Use the *log option* described earlier and check it at least once a week. Be sure you know what areas your children are accessing and how much time they are spending.

More simply stated, set up your system so your children are able to use the Internet as a resource, not as an interactive system. Its greatest value lies in this area and the risks are minimal. If you're not sure how to do this, call your service provider and they will walk you through the steps.

Basic Ground Rules

There is another area of risk: children may provide information on-line that allows someone to send E-mail or other messages that are frightening, harassing, or would allow someone to contact your children or the family. Just as you wouldn't send your child out into a city of 30 million people without supervision and ground rules, you don't want to send your children onto the Internet without limits and ground rules.

If you decide to allow your children to have access to interactive areas, such as the children's chat line, establish clear and nonnegotiable ground rules. Even though these lines are monitored constantly by on-line adult staff, you should be aware that the age range on these chat lines (usually five to fourteen) makes them inappropriate for many preadolescents. Chat lines that are even more age restricted are preferable. A pen pal might be a better choice for younger children. Block all other chat areas.

You should know that on-line services will terminate the accounts of people violating the terms-of-service agreements. You can use this to protect yourself, your children, and other users. If you have any experience that is problematic, notify your on-line service provider immediately. They are responsive.

If you are going to allow your children to participate interactively, I recommend a discussion and that you establish the following ground rules with your children:

1. Never give out your on-line password to anyone. No on-line staff will ever ask for your password.

2. Never reveal personal information, your real name, where you live, your parents' names, telephone number, or where you go to school. Never send pictures of yourself or your family through the Internet.

3. Never continue a conversation that makes you feel uncomfortable, that seems inappropriate, or becomes personal. Just as with the telephone, you can hang up by going to another area of the Internet. Tell your parents about what happened.

4. Always tell your parents about any communication that uses threatening or bad language.

5. Never agree to meet someone. Tell your parents about anyone who makes that suggestion.

6. Do not accept product offers or any other opportunities to send you information through the Internet without your parents' specific approval. Never give your street address to have something mailed.

7. Remember that people on the Internet can be anyone, anywhere. Be cybersmart. Take care of yourself and your family.

As you think about these rules, also think about your children and their vulnerability to adults who have greater knowledge, experience, and powers of persuasion. Asking children to follow these rules may be simple in concept and profoundly difficult for children when the time comes. Consider using the Internet solely for information and resources until your children are in their late teens.

Risk-Taking Behavior on the Internet

Risk-taking behavior is a part of growing up that we address in all areas of child safety. The Internet is no exception. Because the Internet is anonymous, many preadolescent and adolescent children deliberately participate in chat rooms they find titillating. They engage in ongoing conversations with people they describe as "creeps" or "perverts." They tease them and escalate inappropriate discussions. Some even go so far as to set up meetings with these people. This is like "baiting a bear."

Parents can often detect this type of "chat line" activity by using the log, by length of time spent on the Net, by secretiveness when you walk into the room, by lots of friends doing the Net together, or by bragging on the part of the kids about their activities.

This is not acceptable behavior. It is unsafe and inappropriate. This is not a censorship issue. It is not a "you don't trust me" issue. It is a safety issue just like hitchhiking. Discuss this with your children. Be very clear about how you feel and why. Establish a new and clear agreement with your children about the use of the Internet. Contact other parents if it is a group activity. Use the parent control options. Check the log to see if the problem is ongoing. If the problem continues, disconnect the Internet until you can come to a clear consensus and plan for using the Internet in a positive, productive, and safe way.

Monitoring Children's Use of the Internet

It bears repeating that you have to take the lead in protecting your children in the computer age as well as in the park. This means knowing what's going on. On-line services are very responsive to parents and safety concerns. They are making it easier and easier for us to monitor what is going on, where our children are spending their time, and how much money is spent on the Internet.

The Safe Child Book

Get on the Internet yourself. It opens communication between children and parents. Your children want you to know why the Internet is important to them. You need to participate and you need to be the voice for balance. The Internet is more seductive than television. It can be an extraordinary tool and friend or it can be a sinkhole for time and money. As a parent, you need to take the lead and keep it.

Making Exceptions to the Rules

Most parents encourage their children to think for themselves but rarely encourage them to evaluate rules and to make exceptions when they need to. This is a concern because children who feel bound by everyday rules are often unable to get themselves out of problem situations. Children need permission to make exception *to any rule,* if making that exception will keep them safe or allow them to get out of a dangerous situation.

A few examples:

- We teach our children to be polite, then we tell them not to talk to strangers. Which message is stronger when a friendly person walks into the yard and says "Hi"—being polite or not talking to strangers?

- We encourage children to be helpful and we teach them not to take things from strangers. Someone from work drops by and asks your child to give you an important package. Your child doesn't know the person. Would it be okay with you if your children refused the package?

- We teach our children not to keep secrets, then we ask them to. How do children learn when exceptions are okay and when they are not?

- We teach our children the code word. Then we send someone to pick them up without giving them the code word. Will the children get in "trouble" if they refuse to go?

- We teach our children to "mind" without telling them that it's all right to say no if a request seems wrong.

- We teach our children not to lie, without recognizing that lying might be necessary to get them out of a dangerous or compromising situation.

- We teach children not to make too much noise in public places without saying they can "scream like crazy" if they need to.

- We tell them it's all right to hang up on pranksters. Do we then get upset if the prankster they hung up on was an old college friend?

- We tell them not to open the door or accept deliveries when they're home alone. What message do they get if we then grumble all the way to the post office to retrieve an Express Mail letter?

Rules create structure and are crucial to stability, order, and routine in children's lives. While exceptions cannot be taught until you establish the rules, they are important. There are times when children need to be able to make exceptions to the rules. Children who have discretion and responsibility for the rules are better able to make choices that keep them safe.

Being Polite: When Being Rude Means Being Safe

We teach our children to be polite. It is also important to help children develop the ability to judge and decide whether to be polite in specific circumstances. This is true for children of *all* ages. As they grow up, children should have permission to be rude or nonresponsive when *they* feel they need to be. At the same time, we can teach them appropriate behavior. For example, if your child sticks his or her tongue out to express dislike, an instructive response might be: "It's okay that you don't like her. It's not okay for you to stick your tongue out. A better choice would be to ignore her."

One of the most frequent reports I hear from children who have been sexually abused is that they didn't want to hurt the person's feelings or appear rude. **Knowing they have permission to be rude helps children say no to sexual abuse.** It makes it easier for them to ignore or walk away from strangers. It helps free them from the need to please adults to their own detriment.

Lying and Breaking Promises

Most parents teach that lying is totally unacceptable. They might be surprised to hear that this reduces their children's ability to keep themselves safe and to report abuse. For example, I've known many children who were abused and the perpetrator refused to let them go unless they promised not to tell. These children kept their promises. It was not until their parents began to notice changes in their children, which they questioned, that their children revealed the abuse.

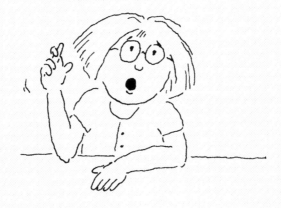

The Safe Child Book

Children must know that it's okay to tell, even when they promised they wouldn't, if they have been threatened or intimidated into promising. This is a difficult exception to teach before about age six. If a child is younger than six, a promise not to tell is the same as a secret. Your children have learned the No More Secrets Rule now and know not to keep secrets, even if they said they would.

It is also essential that your children have the option of lying in order to keep themselves safe or to get out of a risky situation. They have this permission as part of the agreement that they will come and tell you as soon as possible.

Blind Obedience

We need to look at the ways in which we teach our children to be "blindly obedient" to adults and authority figures. Most children do not know they can say no to a policeman, a teacher, a principal, a counselor, a minister, a baby-sitter, or a parent when an inappropriate request is made.

Children need to know that they, and *they alone,* are the judge of the appropriateness of a request. When you cannot be available to help your children make choices, you must give them the ability to make choices for themselves.

Teaching this idea is silly and fun and doesn't interfere with teaching children respect for adults. Use examples such as:

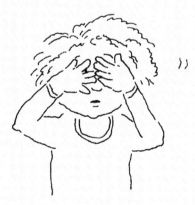

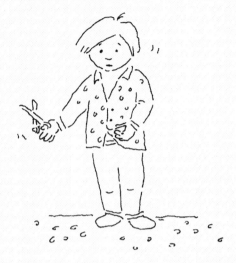

- "What if your teacher said, 'For art today, we're all going to cut little tiny dots out of our shirts and paste them on a piece of paper.'"

    Children will say, "Of course I wouldn't do that. We don't cut holes in our clothes."

- "What if the baby-sitter asked to take a bath with you?"

    Children often say, "I'd say no, the baby-sitter can take a bath when she gets home."

Children already know that their moms and dads and other grown-ups make mistakes. Talk with them about what they would do if Mom or Dad or someone else in the family asks them to do something they know they shouldn't do. Saying no to someone in the family is as important as saying no to people outside the family.

- "What if Dad said you could go across the street to get your ball, but there was a car coming?"

    Children who feel comfortable about Dad making a mistake can say, "I wouldn't go if there was a car coming, even if Dad said okay."

The Safe Child Book

- "What if Mom asked you to keep a secret?"

  If the person who made the rule breaks it, children should feel free to speak up. "Mom, you know we don't keep secrets."

- "What if Mommy's boyfriend asked you to do something you knew was wrong and you were scared to say no because Mommy likes him?"

  Children are at greater risk for abuse with boyfriends and stepfathers. Let your children know they can say no to anyone, that they can come and tell you about what's happened, that you will believe them and that you won't be mad.

The central message underlying all of these stories is this: There isn't anyone in the entire world that your children can't say no to, if they are asked to do something they think is wrong, that could hurt them, or that they know you wouldn't want them to do.

Talk with your children about rules, exceptions, and expectations that allow you to trust one another. Use specific examples and "What If . . ."'s until you're confident they know the difference between blindly doing what they're told and saying no when they need to.

13

Choosing Child Care

Child care has become a major issue for most parents. As the percentage of two-income and single-parent families continues to rise, the need for quality child care has become acute. Leaving your children in someone else's care is, as you well know, one of the most critical decisions you make. Yet, most parents know very little about how to choose and monitor this care.

While it is virtually impossible to remove all the risks, there are guidelines that can help you reduce the vulnerability of your children to abuse by caregivers. The lists I provide here should be added to your overall considerations of any caregiver.

Child care generally falls into several categories:

- Licensed or unlicensed group day care includes any facility that cares for children, whether it has an education program or not.

- Supervised or unsupervised family day care is care in someone's home and often includes the caregiver's own children. Supervision may be provided by a sponsoring referral agency that matches children to specific homes.

- In-home and out-of-home individual care refers to someone who provides care specifically for your children in your home or theirs.

- Finally, there are baby-sitters, who also need special guidelines to help prevent abuse.

While the checklists can be useful, the most important guide you have is your own instinct, your gut reaction to the people and the place where you leave your children. No matter what the checklist says, if your instinct says no, go elsewhere.

Licensed and Unlicensed Group Day Care

Any facility that cares for children, whether licensed or not, should meet stringent standards. These are in addition to any questions and concerns regarding location, cost, education, and other services.

Checklist for Licensed and Unlicensed Centers

The Facility
Is the facility licensed? If not, why not?
What is the general atmosphere?
Is it clean?
Are there separate bathroom facilities for children and adults?

The Staff
Do they seem to enjoy the children? Are they actively interested in what the children are doing?
How do they talk to the children? How much of what is said is corrective ("No," "Stop it") versus instructive.
Is the staff more interested in the children or in talking to you? Are they able to do both?
What are the credentials of the staff?
How long has each person been there?
What are they paid?
Whom do they use for substitutes? What are their credentials and how often are they used?

Are staff members related to one another? If so, how? How long have they worked together? Check all their references.

Do staff members indiscreetly complain about any particular children or families?

Are there any other adults present whose purpose is not clear?

Are there any relatives of staff members who hang around without apparent purpose?

Supervision

How is free time supervised?

What is the adult-to-child ratio?

Is the director always present? If not, who is responsible?

Are the children ever left with only one adult? If so, what happens in an emergency?

How secure is the facility? Could someone come in and pick up a child unnoticed?

Is the playground secure? Are there blind spots where children can't be seen?

Is the playground open to the public?

How are messages handled? Is this a secure system?

Center Activities

Are the children involved in activities? Or do they appear to be looking for something to do?

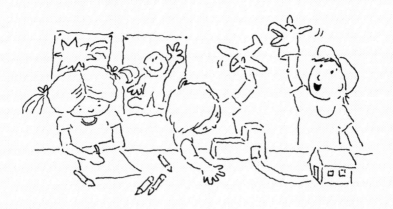

The Safe Child Book

Is there a balance between planned activities and free time?

Are you welcome to drop in at any time? This is extremely important. If not, why not?

Is the children's work displayed? Is it current?

References

Ask for professional references.

Ask for a list of families whose children attend the center, and call them.

Talk with them about the strengths and weaknesses of the center. Find out what problems or concerns they have had. How were they resolved?

Deciding

Trust your instincts. If you're not comfortable with the facility, do not compromise and do not send your children there.

Monitoring

Offer to help on periodic field trips.

Drop in unexpectedly several times a year, including during naptime.

Talk to your children about their day.

Learn to follow up on their answers with additional questions that keep the conversation going. That's where you learn what really happened during their day.

Ask questions like:

"What did you do today?"

"Did anything special happen?"

"Are there any new people at the school?"

"Did you go anywhere special?"

"What did you do at playtime?"

"Did you take a nap?"

If your children tell you about something they didn't like or that made them feel bad, ask more questions, like:

"What does Ms. ——— do?"

"Did you tell her you didn't like it?"

"What did she do or say next?"

"How did you feel when she said that?"

"Would you like me to help by talking to her?"

Let your children know that you can help with problems at the school and demonstrate this by talking with the school even if it's about a small problem. It shows your children that they can call on you for larger problems.

Taking Your Own Concerns Seriously

Immediately act on any concerns you have. Talk to other parents. Find out if they're having similar problems or concerns. Do not be swayed by easy answers or dismissal of your concern by any member of the center staff until you are satisfied with the answer.

Some examples:

What if your child came home with someone else's underwear on and the center says he messed his pants and they borrowed someone else's second pair? Call the other parents.

What if your child comes home with stars on his or her buttocks and upper thigh and the center says it's their way of positively reinforcing potty training? Ask your children what the stars are for.

What if your child comes home with a story about riding to the airport in a van and the center says he or she is confused, they read a story about it. Children know the difference between what they do and what they read about. Ask some other parents.

What if your children come home with stories about people taking pictures of them? The center says that's true and shows you pictures of classroom activities, but you don't feel that's the whole story. Ask other parents about what their children are saying.

All of these situations occurred at one preschool. In each case, the director allayed the concerns of parents with logical explanations. It was only after one child revealed his own abuse and the parents got together that they learned that each of these questions had been a clue to their own children's abuse. As the parents heard only of isolated events, none of them was able to see what was happening.

Paranoia about day care is an ineffective response to child abuse. Careful screening and close monitoring can very effectively protect children. The only child who was not abused at the center referred to above was the one whose mother worked flexible hours and could be expected to show up at any time.

Supervised and Unsupervised Family Day Care

This includes all the people who take children into their home, usually added to their own small children, in a kind of group baby-sitting arrangement. In some cities, this is supervised by a monitoring agency. In others, it is completely unmonitored. Because this is a closed environment, you must be particularly careful when selecting this kind of care.

Checklist for Supervised and Unsupervised Family Day Care

Initial Screening
Do you know the potential caregiver personally?

If not, ask for references and the names of other parents whose children she cares for.

Call the parents and ask about problems, things that annoyed or concerned them. How were they resolved?

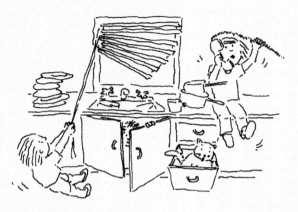

Visiting the Home

What is the general atmosphere?

Is it clean?

Who else lives in the home? Are these people ever there when the children are there?

Is the house large enough to accommodate comfortably the number of children being cared for?

Is the yard secure? For preschoolers, this is essential.

Are the doors easily opened by a small child?

Are there adequate toys and activities for the children?

Does it look as if children live and play there?

Get to Know the Caregiver

Where are the children she is caring for? Where are her own children?

Does she seem to enjoy the children?

How does she talk to the children? How much of what is said is corrective or punitive versus instructive?

What is the maximum number and ages of the children in the home?

What is her education and experience?

Check her past employers, if any.

How does she relate to your children?

Is she more interested in money, hours, and whether you'll ever be late than in your children's needs?

The Safe Child Book

Is there an assistant? Ask all the same questions about the assistant.

How do you feel about the situation?

Ask questions like:

How does she discipline?

What would she do with the children in an emergency?

Do the children play outside alone?

Do they nap? When? Where?

What television programs are the children allowed to watch?

Are you welcome to drop in at any time?

Deciding

Trust your instincts! If you have to sell yourself on this arrangement, find someone else.

Monitoring

Talk to your children. Find out how they feel about being there. (See the "Checklist for Licensed and Unlicensed Centers" earlier in this chapter.)

Drop in unexpectedly from time to time. Change your child's scheduled pickup time every so often.

Immediately act on any concerns you have. Talk to other parents. Do not put up with problems because it would be hard to find another arrangement.

In-Home and Out-of-Home Individual Care

In selecting someone to care for your children in your own home or in theirs, remember that the safety and well-being of your children are being given over to them. What is their experience? Thoroughly check their references and past employers. Notice how they relate to your children. Are they more interested in your children or their own working conditions? How do you feel about them? If you are not comfortable, find someone else. This does not mean that you should hold out for the "perfect" person or that there won't be problems and adjustments. But you must begin with a comfortable base.

Be sure to set specific guidelines and expectations. Do you want someone to care for your children and clean house? Or do you want someone solely to care for your children? Since you are giving the care of your children over to someone else for a period of time, the more they know about your expectations and values about child-rearing, the better job they can do.

Baby-sitters

As dire as the baby-sitter shortage may be, it is important to check out your baby-sitters. Whom else do they sit for? Call those parents. Ask if they had any problems and if they still use this sitter.

Parents commonly leave their children with a baby-sitter and, as they're walking out the door, say, "Now do everything the baby-sitter says." Think about the message implicit in that! It contradicts everything we've been discussing about a child's ability to be responsible and to exercise the skills we are teaching them. The following recommendations will increase the ability of children to keep themselves safe. It also may result in the loss of a baby-sitter or two. I'm sure you'll agree this is a difficult but ultimately worthwhile trade-off in order to protect your children.

When a baby-sitter comes to the house, go over the ground rules for the evening *in the presence of your children.* This includes what they eat, what TV shows and games are allowed, when they go to bed, whether they need a bath—if so, whether they need assistance—do they need help getting ready for bed, do they get snacks, etc.? When this information is covered in the presence of the children, it takes away the baby-sitter's ability to say, "Your parents said ——— and you're really going to get into trouble if they find out you didn't do what I told you to."

Baby-sitters need to be told that you do not permit deviations from these guidelines and that your children will tell you if any are suggested. Tell them also that your children do not keep secrets and will tell you if they are asked to do so. It is important for parents to remember that, first and foremost, the job of a baby-sitter is the care of the children, not being a pal. If the baby-sitter is totally intimidated, it is all right to let her know that you're glad she's there, and it just makes you feel better to give your "standard baby-sitter speech."

Finally, in all child-care arrangements, as in all other situations, the best defense your children have against sexual abuse is the prevention training you give them, your willingness to listen carefully to them, and your ability to ask questions about their concerns.

14

When Children Are Sexually Abused

There is no way to anticipate or remove all the risks to children. In spite of everything we do, some children will be sexually abused. If this happens in your family, another aspect of safety and protection begins. That is, guiding your child through the process of recovery. This is an effort that may conflict with your desire to put it all behind you, with the needs of the system to investigate, and with any attempt to prosecute. This chapter will help you deal with what has happened and suggest ways to advocate for your child.

How Children Tell Us

As you've seen from previous examples, children often do not know how to tell us they have been sexually abused. If they have successfully resisted abuse, they may not know what to do next. There are many reasons for children's hesitancy to talk about what has happened, including their relationship to the abuser, fear of the consequences, or uncertainty about whether or not they will be believed.

This ambivalence can result in some obscure attempts to talk about what happened. For example, one little girl I know said to her father, "Uncle Smitty is ugly." When it was revealed that she had been sexually abused by Uncle Smitty, her father asked why she hadn't told. She adamantly informed him that she *did* tell and cited the day she had said, "Uncle Smitty is ugly."

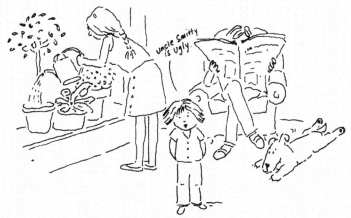

It is important to teach children to say what they mean. It is equally important for parents to learn to listen for what they *mean*, as well as what they say.

Discovering Abuse

More often than not, we discover sexual abuse by observing children's behavior.

Some of the nonverbal signs you can be aware of include:

- Reluctance to go somewhere or be with someone who had previously been okay.

- Inappropriate displays of affection or explicit sexual acts.

- Use of new sexual terms or names for body parts.

- Uncomfortableness with or rejection of typical family affection.

- Sleep problems, including insomnia, nightmares, or refusal to sleep alone.

- Regressive behaviors, including thumb-sucking, bed-wetting, infantile behaviors, or other signs of dependency.

- Extreme clinginess or other signs of fearfulness.

- Depression and withdrawal.

- A sudden change in personality.

- Problems in school.

While all these signs may be related to something other than sexual abuse, they also could be signs of abuse. As you are trying to determine what is wrong, sexual abuse should be one of your considerations. Changes in your child's behavior are signals and may mean your child needs help.

How Should We Respond?

The trauma of children reporting sexual abuse is real, and **one of the most important factors in a child's ability to recover is the reaction of the first person he or she tells.** The foremost concern at that moment should always be calm support.

Do not promise your child that you will do anything specific.

When children report sexual abuse, they should immediately be told:

1. That you believe them and you're glad they told.

2. That they didn't do anything wrong.

3. That the perpetrator shouldn't have done what he or she did.

4. That you will do your best to see that they are not alone with that person again until the problem is resolved.

The Safe Child Book

You may not be able to keep that promise and it adds to their general frustration, disappointment, and sense of betrayal.

Then give yourself some time to think. Parents of abused children are themselves abused. They also feel guilt, rage, and a sense of loss.

If medical assistance is needed immediately for the child, a facility specializing in rape crisis intervention is preferable. They have the necessary training and materials. General anesthesia usually is not recommended to ease the anxiety of the examination. While it makes the physical process easier, it increases the child's sense of helplessness and loss of control.

Whatever medical treatment is required, children should be allowed to participate in the process so they don't feel further victimized by having things "done to them." Let them know where they'll be going. Tell them what will be done and why it is important. Simply saying, "The doctor wants to check you and make sure everything is okay" is a good beginning.

Child sexual abuse is a specialized field. Not everyone is comfortable talking to children about what has happened to them. If your own physician is not familiar with child sexual abuse or doesn't feel comfortable discussing what has happened, ask for a referral to someone who is experienced, who knows what to look for and how to talk to children about what has happened to them.

The emotional damage children experience from sexual abuse is affected by many things. Recovery is easier when children know that you believe them, that they didn't do anything wrong, and that they will not be subject to further abuse. As a parent, you have an opportunity—and a responsibility—to protect your child's emotional well-being during and after the time the abuse is reported.

What About Reporting?

The decision to report sexual abuse is difficult, especially when the perpetrator is a friend, someone well known in the community, or a member of the family. It is important, as you are considering whether or not to report, to remember that the *total* responsibility for the offense lies with the perpetrator. No parent is ever responsible for ruining an abuser's life by reporting.

Children need to participate in the decision to report whenever possible. Do not give your child control of the decision to report. Explain the process. Let your child know he or she will be questioned about what has happened. Ask your child how he or she feels about reporting the abuser. Acknowledge how frightening the entire situation is.

Explain the importance of reporting so your child will not be abused again and so other children will not be abused. I find that most children want the offender to get help and also want to protect other children from future abuse.

Your decision to report needs to include consideration of your child's safety and ability to recover. It also needs to include a consideration of other children. The average pedophile abuses over seventy children in his or her "career" of offending. Your child probably was not the first nor will he or she be the last.

Many parents—motivated by outrage, disbelief, and a fear of falsely accusing—want to talk to the accused abuser before reporting. I strongly discourage this. Perpetrators are very convincing and will only confuse the situation by their denial. Call the child abuse hotline, your local child protective services agency, social services, or police department. You do not need evidence or anything other than your child's story. The job of investigating belongs to the system.

To get more information on how to report abuse in your state you can call the

NATIONAL CHILD ABUSE HOTLINE: 1-800-4ACHILD

They will direct you to the proper agency.

If you want to consult someone before reporting to help you decide whether or not you want to report, it is important that you

The Safe Child Book

understand the mandatory reporting law. In all fifty states and the District of Columbia, professionals (that is, anyone who works in a position of trust with children, including doctors, nurses, teachers, social workers) are required by law to report all suspected cases of child abuse or neglect. In addition, therapists, rabbis, priests, and ministers are required to report. This means that the professional you consult will be bound by law to report the case. Parents who are not aware of this law can be devastated by an unexpected police or social services investigation.

What Happens Next?

Once a decision to report is made, parents need to retain as much control of the process as possible. Children also need to be informed about what is going to happen, and they should have input in the decisions that are being made, if they are able to do so. Contrary to widely held belief, we do not protect children when we keep them in the dark. Children who have been abused have a right to be part of the decision-making process after their abuse.

Parents need to seek out the best and most experienced people in the field. They must be willing to go to higher levels if they are dissatisfied with the way they or their children are being treated. It cannot be assumed that everyone is adequately trained or able to be effective in every situation.

After a report is made, children are often interviewed repeatedly. As a parent, you have the right to question this process, to request that interviews be audiotaped, videotaped, and consolidated to prevent what professionals call "revictimization" of your child. If your child is to testify, be sure he or she understands what will happen, what kinds of questions will be asked, and what is expected. Finally, be sure your child understands that the perpetrator will be present.

While I believe that we must report, that we must find better ways to allow children to testify, that child abuse must be treated as a serious crime, the sad truth is, it is not. Sex abusers have the

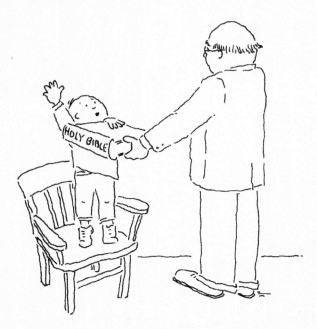

lowest conviction rate of any crime. Only one in every sixty reported cases results in a conviction. Those convicted serve an average of less than twelve months in jail.

This is changing. Treatment programs for abusers are expanding, innovative programs are requiring treatment rather than incarceration, public demand is resulting in stiffer sentences for repeat offenders, new and creative legislation is being passed that recognizes the special nature of crimes against children. It is not enough, but every case that is reported brings closer the day when sexual abuse of children will no longer be an ever-present possibility.

Is Therapy Necessary?

Parents often consider therapy unnecessary for child sexual abuse victims, particularly for boys. Parents say things to me like "Let's let him forget it. He doesn't seem upset to me." **Do not be fooled. Everything we know about child sexual abuse tells us that its effects are long-lasting and devastating.**

The Safe Child Book

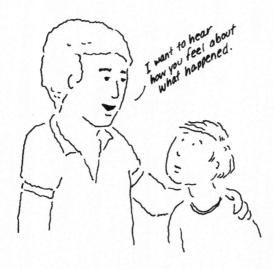

It is not true that children forget if the adults around them do not talk about it or allow them to talk about it. Sexual abuse incidents are intensely real for children, whether they talk about it or not.

One of the most important elements in a child's recovery is the placing of responsibility where it lies—with the perpetrator. Parents aren't the best ones to communicate this message to children because children expect their parents to stick up for them. A professional can be very important to the

The degree of impact sexual abuse has on a child is determined by several factors:

1. The type and severity of the abuse.

2. The relationship of the perpetrator to the child.

3. How long the abuse continued.

4. The reaction of the people the child tells.

5. Support available to the child to recover fully.

child's ability to resolve the many issues that arise after sexual abuse.

There are now many professionals who can provide the necessary therapeutic intervention, who know how to work with children who have been sexually abused. They can help children to understand that what happened wasn't their fault, and that they didn't do anything wrong. Through treatment, children can reestablish their sense of trust with adults and themselves. This may take two weeks or two years, depending on the child and the abuse. But it is remarkable to watch children recover from the subtle and profound effects of abuse.

15

Being a Responsible Adult

As adults learn more about child abuse and abduction, they begin to evaluate their behavior toward other people's children and even their own. They ask questions like "Am I being too affectionate?" One common impulse is to withdraw, to be less playful and affectionate with children, lest something be misinterpreted or misunderstood. While this is an understandable reaction, holding back is *not* an effective way to respond to this problem.

Rules for Responsible Strangers

We know who we are; children don't. We know we are safe, harmless, and well-intentioned, and yet we look the same to a child as an offender might look. It is important to be friendly, but we've got to balance that friendliness with a recognition of the realities for children.

As strangers, we, too, must follow the stranger rules. We need to **avoid starting up casual conversations with children who are not with an adult.** This means that we shouldn't ask children who are alone for directions, for the time, or for assistance, or to chat with them about their dog, a toy, or whatever.

While we know we represent no threat, those same comments or requests can be made by the "nicest people in the world" who later turn out to be dangerous. **Children can't read minds, so they have no way of knowing whom they should**

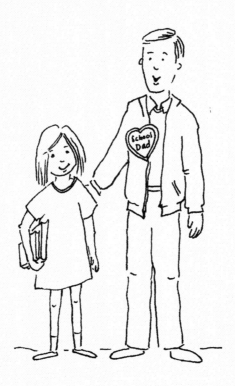

talk to. They have to follow the stranger rules with all strangers, even you.

Here are some situations where we should follow the rules:

- What if a child approaches you in the park and wants to talk? A parent is present, but not really watching. One option is to ask the child if Mom or Dad said it was okay for him to talk to you. If not, tell him he should get permission before talking to you because he doesn't know you.

- What if you are giving samples or treats away as a part of your job or at a school event? Always ask parents if it's all right to give the item to their children. This reinforces the parents' role as protectors when they are with their children.

The Safe Child Book

- What if you need to drop something off for a business associate whose children you do not know? Don't ask the children to take the item. Instead, deliver it directly to the parent.

With older children, it is generally all right to make small talk in a public setting when other people are around. It is not as appropriate in a more isolated setting. You should let children take the lead in terms of what is *their* comfort level. Be sensitive to small signs that suggest children are uncomfortable, and stop talking.

I know this seems restrictive and creates uncertainty about how we should behave with children. As often as I speak about this, I still have to monitor myself to follow the rules with children I don't know. But when I see children who follow the rules with me, I know they are less vulnerable to the "friendly" stranger who might hurt them.

Lost Children

On the other hand, children sometimes need help. When they do, you should stop and help. You can do this in such a way that your intervention is not suspect and the child is protected from exploitation by someone else.

For example, if you see a lost child in a store, approach her, ask if she is lost and escort her to the front of the store, where a clerk or manager can page her parents. Do not pick the child up and carry her. Hold her hand and walk with her, telling her where you're taking her and why. If possible, do not leave her until she is reunited with her parents. It is not appropriate to take her to get a cola or to wander around the store looking for her parents. You need to protect yourself even as you protect the child.

Helping lost children is an excellent opportunity to teach them what they should do the next time they're in a similar situation. Children are very receptive when they're lost, as are their parents, to hearing about strategies that you've found work with your own children.

Children We Know

The suggestions for teaching prevention of sexual abuse to your own children can be applied to other children. For example, when you are greeted with a big hug from the child of a friend, it feels terrific. If the child moves away, even though you'd like another hug, the best response is "That was a nice hug. Thank you for letting me know you were ready to get down."

For example, if you're stroking your nephew's hair and he asks you to stop or wiggles away, you can say, "I didn't know you don't like that. Thanks for telling me to stop. If I forget, you can remind me."

What if the child of a friend is consistently shy and her dad keeps encouraging her to talk and be affectionate with you because you're a friend? You might say to the dad, "I'm really *your* friend right now, not hers."

Children show us more often than they tell us what they like and don't like. We can give them permission to speak up and let them know that we don't feel rejected just because they ask us not to do something. Experiencing this with a variety of adults greatly strengthens their ability to use the prevention techniques.

Child Advocacy

In teaching prevention, we ask children to tell us what is happening to them. Do we listen? What if a child whispers to us, "This man won't let me see my mommy"? What do we say? How do we start? Do we dismiss it as the active imagination of a playful child? Even if we say something, the adult may respond with "Oh, she's always saying things like that to get attention." Do we walk away? Do we report it? Do we tag along to get the license number of their car?

If we see a screaming child being carried from a store, what do we think? Most adults see a temper tantrum. Children, by the way, see this as a child in trouble with no one helping, not even Mom and Dad. What do we do? Are we able to ask what's happening to the child? One option would be to approach and say, "Are you giving your mother a hard time?" If the child responds with "This is not my mother, she's taking me away," the situation changes dramatically.

How often do we remain silent, not wishing to interfere, afraid we will falsely accuse someone? How does fear of the consequences of our intrusion stop us? There are no simple answers, but the impact of courageous intervention is unmistakable in the following story.

There was a woman sitting at the back of a commercial plane who repeatedly slapped her five-year-old for crying. The passengers were unavoidably aware of the situation. After about thirty minutes, a lady a few rows forward stood up, turned around, and said, "If you touch her again, I'll come and take her away from you." Everyone broke out into applause and the child was not touched again during the flight.

While this child may have been beaten more severely later because of the embarrassment to her mother, the undeniable fact remains that the child discovered that the world is not silent in the face of her abuse. This example is significant because the universal comment of abused children is "I couldn't understand why no one said or did anything. I thought grown-ups just didn't care." The child on the plane now knows that there are people in the world who do care and who will help her. That, in and of itself, will make it easier for her to ask for help in the future.

I admit it can be very hard to find the courage to speak up so forthrightly. **Each of us must do what we can do to support children, to report what's done to them.** The law protects people who report suspected child abuse and neglect. You have the right to remain anonymous and you cannot be sued or found liable for damages unless it can be proven that you were malicious and deliberate in filing a false report.

We are teaching children to take care of themselves when they're by themselves. At the same time, children need our care, too. If each of us were an advocate for each of the children in our lives, those we know and those we don't, the abuse of children would significantly diminish. This is not simple or easy. It is, however, a process, a beginning, by which we can reduce the isolation and victimization of children.

When we speak up for children, they learn to speak up for themselves. That is the challenge.

16

Safety in Schools

Just as parents need to be advocates for their own and other children, schools need to be very clear about their role in the protection of children. As obvious as this statement seems, it is an area that is not addressed sufficiently by too many schools. I have served as an expert witness in cases involving schools that took the position that children were not their responsibility once they had been dropped off at school, that their responsibility began when the morning bell rang. This is clearly not a position of advocacy and shared responsibility.

Children spend six to ten hours a day at school, depending on their participation in before- and after-school programs. This means that a significant part of their lives are separate from your ability to protect them. This chapter will look at some areas in which schools can both assess their current practices and policies and consider changes.

Screening and Training of Employees

All staff (including janitors, cafeteria workers, playground monitors, and professional staff) should be fingerprinted and checked through the Central Registry for Child Abuse and state and local police files for a history of child abuse or other criminal convictions. Individuals with a history of child abuse should not be hired for any position.

All staff should receive training in recognizing signs of child abuse and neglect. All should be informed about the mandatory reporting law and reporting requirements of the school and school district.

Ask your school about its hiring policies and practices, specifically in the areas of background checks and school procedures for reporting suspected abuse.

Child Abuse Reporting

The mandatory reporting law requires any staff member who has reason to know or suspect that a child has been subjected to abuse or neglect, or who has observed a child being subjected to circumstances or conditions that are or could result in abuse or neglect, to report it. In some cases, school policy requires that the report be made to the administration. In some cases, the report can be made directly to the child abuse hotline. All employees should understand that failure to make such a report is a crime. You have every right to ask for a copy of the school's child abuse reporting policies and procedures.

Playground Security

Supervision of children who are dropped at school prior to the time school opens is the subject of an ongoing battle for most schools and parents. In some communities, this is a particularly adversarial situation resulting in calls to the police and social services when children are dropped off early. In other communities, schools have responded, often with parental participation, and now provide before-school programs as early as 7:00 A.M. that include snacks and planned activities.

The same situation exists after school. Some schools ask all children to leave the building, close their doors thirty minutes after school ends, and take no responsibility for children remaining in the area. Other schools have after-school programs that again provide snacks and supervision until 5:00 or 6:00 P.M. These pro-

Example of Ideal Parent/School Communication
(Posted in Office of School and Provided in Writing
for Every New Parent)

WHAT YOU NEED TO KNOW ABOUT CHILD ABUSE AND NEGLECT

All our staff receive training in recognizing signs of physical or sexual abuse or neglect in children.

Any staff member who has reasonable cause to know or suspect that a child has been subjected to abuse or neglect, or who has observed a child being subjected to circumstances or conditions that constitute or could result in abuse or neglect, shall immediately make a written report to the director. The school is required by law to report any such incidents to the Department of Social Services.

We require all our staff to be fingerprinted for investigation by the Central Bureau of Investigation and to be cleared by the Central Registry for Child Abuse.

If a parent at any time suspects child abuse or neglect on the part of our staff, or by any other person visiting the school, we ask you to please inform us immediately and to report your concerns to the Department of Social Services.

We have provided you with a letter detailing how you can report suspected child abuse or neglect, issued by the Department of Social Services.

If you have any questions regarding the above policy, please feel free to discuss your concerns with us.

grams are often run by parents who are paid a small fee by parents using the service.

Schools cannot ignore the work requirements and child-care

dilemmas of today's parents. They cannot take a position of blaming. They need to confront the problem and work with parents to create a solution that takes care of the children. This is always doable if there is a commitment on the part of everyone to do what is right for the children.

Parents should not be daunted by claims of liability or other legal arguments against using school buildings. These are not the issue. The issue is the school's willingness to get involved in meeting the needs of the community, parents, and children. Working together, this can be done.

Walking to School and the Bus

Children need to walk in pairs or groups to school or to the bus. If they cannot, parents should walk with their children, pair them up with older children, or drive their children. Single chil-

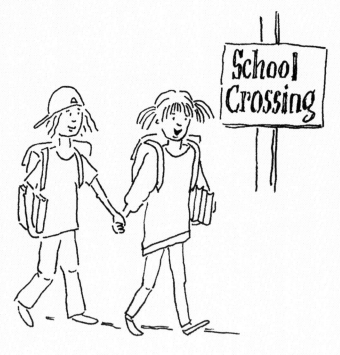

dren on the street are more vulnerable. Don't let your kids tell you it's a matter of trust or treating them like a baby. It's a matter of doing your job as a parent to protect your kids.

Some school districts have changed their bus routes to ensure that single children are not waiting for a bus or being dropped off alone. Don't be shy about talking with your school about bus routes and supervision. By the way, bus drivers should also be subject to background searches, even if they are not school employees but are contracted through another company.

Neighborhood Watch

If you live in a community where children walk to school, you should have a neighborhood watch or safe house program. Your local police department can assist you and the school to put something in place. This designates specific homes on each block as well as community businesses that will help children in need of assistance.

Businesses are particularly helpful. In the case of neighborhood homes, these people are never screened, so I suggest that children not enter these homes or use them unless it is an emergency or they have been frightened by something that has happened on the way to or from school. Parents should take a walk with their children and visit each safe house between home and school.

Parents on Patrol

One school district I've worked with developed Parents on Patrol (POP), in which one parent patrols each block, in a POP vest, to ensure the safety of children walking to school. They worked out a schedule in which parents worked one morning and one afternoon per week on the blocks used by children on the way to school.

Perimeter Issues

School playgrounds should be fenced. Areas that cannot be seen by supervising school personnel should not be used by children. Fences should be in good repair with no areas that could injure children.

Children should never be on the playground without active supervision. A cluster of adults chatting on the playground is not supervision.

If your school is inadequately staffed, perhaps parents can work from the model being used at a neighborhood school in Denver. The first-grade parents have a schedule to assist with recess and lunch duty. Each parent who is able to help comes once or twice a month to provide additional playground supervision for the children during morning recess and lunch. There are about five hundred other children on the playground, but the parents' job is to help supervise the first-grade class. As this model has evolved, most parents end up acting as aides in the classroom for the morning. This has been a real contribution to the classroom and to teacher-parent communication—and the kids love the special day when their parents come and stay.

Playground Equipment

Take a walk out to your school's playground. Equipment that is not in good repair is a preventable accident waiting to happen. Speak to your school about it. If the repairs cannot be made immediately, be persistent about having one of two things happen. Either rope off the area so children cannot play there until the equipment is repaired or get a group of parents together on a Saturday and fix up the playground to a safe level.

Locked Buildings

Some smaller schools, particularly preschools that do not have full-time front-door staff, keep their buildings locked to prevent people walking in unannounced. Some schools use a pass system, much like a parking pass, which opens the door for the parent. Others use an intercom connected to the office. For some, a doorbell is sufficient. Look at the physical layout of your school and discuss what security measures seem appropriate.

Identification of Guests in the Building

It is important for children and staff to know who's in the school. One way to identify unknown people in the building is to use ID tags or other identification. One school used a picture of their mascot on a string. Any guest in the building was given one to wear when he or she checked in with the office. This type of system has two benefits. It makes sure that people check in with the office. Secondly, it lets children know who has permission to be in the building.

Going to and from Buildings on a Campus

Some schools have a number of buildings on a campus. Children often move between them alone or in groups. Go to the school and hang out for a few hours. Are there children wandering around who didn't get where they were going and who are unsupervised? How does the school know who belongs on the campus and who doesn't? Is there a check-in procedure for people entering the campus?

Pickups During and After School

Schools are very aware in theory about not releasing children to anyone other than the persons designated to pick them up. In practice, I have found schools to be extremely lax about this. Most have no idea who picks up children after school. Go to your child's school early one afternoon and watch what happens after school. Then talk about this with your child.

If your life situation is such that this is a particular concern for you, set up a more concrete pickup plan for your children— for example, picking them up in the office. Set up a code word that ensures that no one who is unauthorized to pick up your child is able to do so. Check and make sure that the code word is actually workable. Require that the school check the ID of anyone picking up the child using the code word. Be sure your child also understands the rules in case the staff fails to follow the guidelines.

Absences and the Call System

Every child should be accounted for every morning. Schools should request that parents call the school when the child will not be in school. Once attendance is taken, the parents of any child not accounted for should be called. This accomplishes two important things. In the event of an abduction, the parents know there is a problem shortly after school starts, not several hours later. Second, if the child is truant, parents are notified immediately.

In many schools, parents assist in this process as well. Parents can work as little as one day during the school year making these follow-up calls.

Substitutes

Remember the days when you came to school, walked into your classroom, and saw a new name on the blackboard? Then a total stranger said, "Hi, I'm your substitute teacher for today." A better approach is having a substitute teacher introduced to the children by a member of the staff. This takes only a minute, but establishes an immediate connection for the children.

Field Trips

It's tough to maintain an accurate head count during field trips. Be sure that your school has a system for field trips so children know what adults they are with and so adults know all children are accounted for.

At one school, parents provided the school with laminated tags on plastic lanyards for every child and staff person. The tag included the school name and phone number and, on the other side, in small letters, the child's name and class. Extras were provided for parents working on field trips. This made it easy to identify who belonged with the group and saved the teacher having to make name tags for every field trip. It also prevented children walking around with their names emblazoned across their chests.

Head-counting is part of field trips. Before leaving or entering any area, heads should be counted to be certain every child is present. This is not just the teacher's job. You can do it, too.

Prevention Programs in the Schools

You've probably discovered that children often take things they hear in school more seriously than what they hear at home. The school is a critical partner in prevention of child abuse. Ask about a child abuse prevention curriculum in your school system. Do they have a program that is age-appropriate, role-play based, and that gives children lots of opportunities to think about and practice prevention techniques without being fearful or explicit? If you would like to introduce your school to the Safe Child Program, share this book with them or request a brochure from the Coalition for Children (see pages 161–62).

Working Together

I'm sure you noted how many times in this chapter I have suggested parental participation in the school's safety efforts. This is partly practical and partly designed to increase parent/school dialogue about children's well-being.

It takes all of us to create a safer place for our children. That's our job. When we fail, the training and techniques provided in this book will maximize your children's ability to protect themselves.

Appendix: The Safe Child Program

The Safe Child Program is a comprehensive curriculum for the prevention of child abuse. It contains all the key components that have been identified as essential to a comprehensive prevention of child abuse program, including:

- teacher training to ensure consistent presentation of the program;

- parental involvement to enhance understanding and support of program goals;

- multiracial and multicultural (parent and child materials are available in English, Spanish, Creole, and French);

- positive, nonexplicit approach that respects the needs of children and families;

- program initiation at the preschool level with annual, age-appropriate development of the concepts and skills;

- multisession instruction, five to ten sessions each year of the program;

- videotapes to guarantee the accurate introduction and modeling of the concepts to the children;

- well-scripted classroom role-playing to develop individual mastery of safety skills;

- emphasis on life skills that have been shown to enable children to utilize prevention skills; and

- ongoing evaluation and updating of the program.

Presented in a preschool-to-third-grade series, it teaches children to think for themselves, to speak up for themselves, and to know when and how to ask for help. In nearly a decade of ongoing evaluation, the Safe Child Program has demonstrated clearly that it reduces children's risk of abuse and enhances their personal safety.

To learn more about this curriculum, write or call:

Coalition for Children
P.O. Box 6304
Denver, CO 80206
1-800-320-1717

Or visit our Web page on the Internet: http://www.safechild.org

Notes on Sources

Page

Chapter 1: The Basics . . .

11 *"Child abuse and neglect in the United States":* U.S. Department of Health and Human Services, Administration for Children and Families, U.S. Advisory Board on Child Abuse and Neglect, *The Continuing Child Protection Emergency: A Challenge to the Nation* (Washington, D.C.: U.S. Government Printing Office, April 1993).

11 *Over 3 million cases of child abuse:* Deborah Daro, D.S.W., Director, and Karen McCurdy, M.A., Principal Analyst, *Current Trends in Child Abuse Reporting and Fatalities: The Results of the 1995 Annual Fifty State Survey,* prepared by the National Center on Child Abuse Prevention Research, a program of the National Committee for Prevention of Child Abuse.

11 *Eighty-five to 90 percent of sexual abuse:* Diana E. H. Russell, *Sexual Exploitation, Rape, Child Sexual Abuse, and Workplace Harassment,* Sage Library or Social Research 155 (Newbury Park, Calif.: Sage Publications, 1984).

11 *One in every four girls and one in every six boys:* Alfred Kinsey et al., *Sexual Behavior of the Human Female* (Philadelphia: W. B. Saunders, 1953).

12 *Approximately one-third of sexual abuse cases:* National Center on Child Abuse and Neglect, *Study of National Incidence and Prevalence of Child Abuse and Neglect: 1988* (Washington, D.C.: U.S. Department of Health and Human Services, 1988).

12 *Ninety-five percent of child abusers:* J. R. Conte, S. Wolf, and T. Smith, "What Sexual Offenders Tell Us About Prevention Strategies," *Child Abuse and Neglect* 13, no. 2 (1989): 143–47.

12 *Eighty percent of substance abusers:* Daytop conference, New York City, 1988, interview, 1988.

12 *Eighty percent of runaways:* Denver Police Department: conference, 1985; interview, 1986. Also, J. Baumeister, Franklin County Children Services "Unruly Youth" Program, Columbus, Ohio, March 1980, cited in Victoria Kepler, *One in Four: Handling Child Sexual Abuse—What Every Professional Should Know* (Privately published, 1984).

12 *Seventy-eight percent of our prison population:* Nicholas Groth, Oklahoma City, conference, 1986; interview, 1993.

12 *Ninety-five percent of prostitutes:* Conte et al., "What Sexual Offenders Tell Us."

13 *Ninety-two percent of all teachers believe:* Joan Cole Duffell, "National Teacher Survey Reveals Wide Gap Between Policy and Practice in Abuse Prevention," *Prevention Notes* (Seattle, Wash.: 1990).

13 *Ninety percent of the public believe:* Duffell, "National Teacher Survey Reveals Wide Gap."

13 *It is now evident that "one-shot" efforts:* Ian Gentles and Elizabeth Cassidy, *Evaluating the Evaluators: Child Sexual Abuse Prevention* (Toronto: Human Life Institute, 1988). Also, Sherryll Kraizer, Susan S. Witte, and George E. Fryer, Jr., "Child Sexual Abuse Programs: What Makes Them Effective in Protecting Children," *Children Today,* September–October 1989.

14 *Developmentally appropriate materials:* Deborah Daro, "Prevention—Replicating Child Abuse Prevention Programs: A Word of Caution," *APSAC Advisor,* Spring 1991. Also, S. Wurtele, D. Saslawsky, C. Miller, S. Marrs, and J. Britcher, "Teaching Personal Safety Skills for Potential Prevention of Sexual Abuse: A Comparison of Treatments," *Journal of Consulting and Clinical Psychology* 54 (1986): 688–92.

14 *It is compellingly obvious:* National Center on Child Abuse and Neglect, *Study of National Incidence and Prevalence of Child Abuse.*

14 *Preschool appears to be:* Kraizer, Witte, and Fryer, "Child Sexual Abuse Prevention Programs." Also, Sherryll Kraizer, George E. Fryer, and Marilyn Miller, "Programming for Preventing Sexual Abuse and Abduction: What Does It Mean When It Works?," *Child Abuse* (Journal of the Child Welfare League of America), January–February 1988.

14 *Prevention education:* Daro, "Prevention—Replicating Child Abuse Prevention Programs." Also, George E. Fryer, Sherryll Kraizer, and Thomas Miyoshi, "Measuring Actual Reduction of Risk to Child Abuse: A New Approach," and ibid., "Measuring Children's Retention of Skills to Resist Stranger Abduction: Use of the Simulation Technique," *Child Abuse and Neglect* 11 (1987). Also, Kraizer, Witte, and Fryer, "Child Sexual Abuse Prevention Programs," and Kraizer, Fryer, and Miller, "Programming for Preventing Sexual Abuse and Abduction."

14 *It is not necessary for programming to be explicit:* Kraizer, Witte, and Fryer, "Child Sexual Abuse Prevention Programs"; Kraizer, Fryer, and Miller, "Programming for Preventing Sexual Abuse and Abduction"; and Sherryll Kraizer, "Rethinking Prevention," *Child Abuse and Neglect* 10 (1986).

14 *The opportunity to apply concepts:* Kraizer, "Rethinking Prevention"; Fryer, Kraizer, and Miyoshi, "Measuring Actual Reduction of Risk to Child Abuse"; Fryer, Kraizer, and Miyoshi, "Measuring Children's Retention of Skills to Resist Stranger Abduction": Kraizer, Witte, and Fryer, "Child Sexual Abuse Prevention Programs"; and Kraizer, Fryer, and Miller, "Programming for Preventing Sexual Abuse and Abduction."

Chapter 9: Staying Alone

88 *In a nationwide research effort:* Sherryll Kraizer, "Children in Self-Care: A New Perspective," *Child Welfare,* November 1990.

Index

abduction:
> best defense against, 19, 85, 86
> and older children, 79
> and strangers, 65, 72
> and "What If . . ." game, 30
> "What if they get me anyway?,"
> 85

absence, from school, 158

abuse, *see* child abuse; sexual
abuse

abusers, *see* offenders

accidents, and self-care, 97–98

adults:
> blind obedience to, 44, 123–25
> and bullying, 108
> caretaking, presence of, 77, 79
> mistakes made by, 124–25
> mixed messages from, 53–55,
> 120–21
> permission from, 80, 146
> physical power of, 32
> respect for, 44
> responses of, 55–58
> rules for, 62–63, 145–50
> support and help from, 99,
> 142–43, 145–50
> *see also* parents

affection, and touching, 55–56

after-school programs, 152–53

alone, *see* self-care

anonymity, and Internet, 114, 118

answering machines, 93

answering the door, 95–96

answering the telephone, 92–95

anxiety, *see* fear

Arm's Reach Plus rule, 72–76
> and circle of safety, 72
> defined, 72
> and embarrassment, 76
> and role-play, 74
> for seven years old and older, 76
> and Stand Up, Back Up, and Run
> To . . . game, 74–75
> for three- to seven-year-olds,
> 73–75

assertiveness, 52

attention, attracting, 85

baby-sitters, 134–35

bad guys vs. good guys, 66–68, 145

"badness," body parts and, 48

betrayal, in sexual abuse, 41–42

blame, avoidance of, 106

blind obedience, 44, 123–25

body, ownership of, 50–51

body language, 52

body parts:
> and "badness," 48
> and masturbation, 48, 49
> new names for, 47, 137

body parts (*cont.*)
    private parts, 52–53
    and touching, 50–51
    understanding of, 48
boyfriends, as abusers, 43–44
bribery, as offender's tool, 45, 60, 66
bullies, 100–108
    compassion lacked by, 101
    forms of, 101
    and prevention, 104–8
    provocation of, 102
    and victims, 101, 102
    of your child, 102–5
    your children as, 105–6
bus, school, 154–55

call system, in schools, 158
campus, school, 157
candy, from strangers, 79–82
caretaking adults, *see* adults; child
    care; parents
Central Registry for Child Abuse,
    151
child abuse:
    age of onset, 14
    best defense against, 19
    Central Registry for, 151
    national hotline, 140
    reporting of, 141, 152
    and social problems, 12
    statistics about, 11–13
    and therapy, 142–44
    see also sexual abuse
child advocacy, 148–50
child care, 126–35
    activities in, 128–29
    baby-sitters, 134–35
    caregiver in, 132–33
    categories of, 126–27
    concerns about, 130–31
    facilities for, 127
    family day care, 131–33
    group day care, 127–31
    individual care, 133–34
    initial screening of, 131
    monitoring of, 129–30, 133

references for, 129
staff of, 127–28
supervision of, 128
visits to, 132
children:
    abilities of, 18
    abuse of and by, 44–45
    alone, 69–70, 88–99; *see also* self-
        care
    as bullies, 100–108
    decision making by, 8–9, 40,
        55–56, 63
    egocentricity of, 37
    empowerment of, 14
    expectations of, 83
    generalization by, 18–19, 35, 69
    instincts of, 21–22, 84–85
    judgment of, 19
    known to us, 148
    letting go of, 24
    names of, 78–79
    as offenders, 44–45
    older, 79
    partnership with, 86
    point of view of, 66–67
    responsibility of, 18, 69–70, 86
    rural, 89
    and secrecy, 61–62
    setting guidelines for, 8
    speaking up, 18, 40, 52, 56, 148,
        149–50
    suburban, 89
    touching of, *see* touching
    urban, 89
    vulnerability of, 8, 31–32, 44, 79,
        117
    window into minds of, 26–27
circle of safety, 72
code word, 84, 117, 158
coercion, emotional, 60
common ground, establishment of,
    70–71
communication:
    body language in, 52
    child abuse hotline, 140
    Don't Talk to Strangers, 77–79

hesitancy about, 136–37
on Internet, *see* Internet
learning skills of, 77
mixed messages in, 53–55,
    120–21
and preteens, 32–33
and prevention, 58, 63–64
role-play in, 74
school-parent, 153
of support and help, 142–43
telephone answering, 92–95
see also "I'm going to tell"; telling
compassion, lack of, 101
computers, *see* Internet
control:
of Internet activities, 115–16,
    118–19
loss of, 42
of telephone calls, 95

day care, *see* child care
decision making, by children, 8–9,
    40, 55–56, 63
defense, aspects of, 19, 86; *see also*
    prevention
disruption, in sexual abuse, 46
doctor, playing, 47, 48–49
Don't Go Anywhere with a
    Stranger, 82–83
Don't Take Things from Strangers,
    79–82
eight years and older, 81–82
three- to seven-year-olds, 80–81
Don't Talk to Strangers, 77–79
door, answering, 95–96

egocentricity, of children, 37
eight years and older, Don't Take
    Things from Strangers rule for,
    81–82
E-mail, on Internet, 111, 116
embarrassment, of preteens, 32,
    56–57, 76
emergencies, and self-care, 97–98
emotional coercion, 60
employees, school, 151–52

empowerment, of children, 14
E-zines, on Internet, 111–12

family:
disruption of, 46
and incest, 43, 64
and runaways, 64
see also parents
family day care, 131–33
caregiver in, 132–33
deciding on, 133
initial screening of, 131
monitoring of, 133
visiting, 132
fantasy vs. reality, 32, 46–47
father/daughter incest, 43
fear:
avoidance of, 29
and feelings, 85
and generalization, 35
and prevention, 67
projection of, 35
safety without, 17–19
and self-care, 97
and sexual abuse, 46
and telling, 63
"What if they get me anyway?," 85
feeling funny inside (instincts),
    21–22, 84–85
field trips:
head-counting and, 159
ID tags for, 79, 159
fingerprinting, of school employ-
    ees, 151–52
fires, and self-care, 97–98
freedom of movement, 32, 86
friendship, as offender's tool, 45, 66

games:
Stand Up, Back Up, and Run
    to . . ., 74–75
"What if . . . ," *see* "What If . . ."
    game
generalization, 18–19
and fear, 35
and strangers, 69

genitals, *see* body parts
getting lost, 28–29, 147–48
good guys vs. bad guys, 66–68, 145
grooming process, of offenders, 45
group day care, 127–31
    activities in, 128–29
    concerns about, 130–31
    deciding on, 129
    facilities for, 127
    monitoring of, 129–30
    references for, 129
    staff of, 127–28
    supervision of, 128
grown-ups, *see* adults; parents
guilt:
    misbehavior and, 37–38
    sexual abuse and, 46

help, resources for, 99
home alone, *see* self-care
hotline, child abuse, 140
household noises, 97

"I don't care," 60
ID tags:
    for field trips, 79, 159
    in school, 157
"I'm going to tell," 58–59
    and emotional coercion, 60
    offenders' response to, 60
    and secrets, 62
    vs. tattling, 59
    whom to tell, 63–64
"I'm watching you" telephone calls,
    95
incest, 43, 64
independence:
    freedom of movement, 86
    preteens' wish for, 32
individual care, in-home and out-
    of-home, 133–34
instincts, of children, 21–22, 84–85
Internet, 109–19
    access to, 111
    alarm clock, 113
    anonymity of, 114, 118

balance with other elements of
    life, 112
blocking parts of, 115–16
bulletin board services, 115
cap on bill for, 113
chat lines on, 111, 115, 116, 118
and child-driven learning, 112
costs of, 112–13
described, 109–11
E-mail, 111, 116
E-zines, 111–12
ground rules for, 116–17
instant messages, 115
internal log in, 113, 116, 118
kids on, 112–13
log of on-line time on, 113
monitoring child's use of, 118–19
news groups, 115
options for, 113
parental control of, 115–16,
    118–19
parts of, 111–12
passwords on, 117
pen pals and, 111, 116
and personal meetings, 117
as resource, 116
risks of, 113–15
risk-taking behavior on, 118
safety on, 115–16, 118
strangers on, 114–15, 117
time on, 113
trust and, 114–15
and vulnerability, 117
Web, 112

judgment, of children, 19

karate mentality, 32
kindergartners:
    Arm's Reach Plus rule for, 73–75
    and prevention, 56
    and "What If . . ." game, 31

language, bad, and Internet,
    115–16, 117
learning, child-driven, 112

listening:
   and positive reinforcement, 63
   telling and, 63–64
lost children, 28–29, 147–48
lying:
   about sexual abuse, 46–47
   and safety, 122–23

make-believe vs. reality, 32, 46–47
mandatory reporting law, 141, 152
masturbation, 48, 49
media, abuse reported in, 47
misbehavior, and guilt, 37–38
movement, freedom of, 32, 86

names, strangers' knowledge of,
   78–79
national child abuse hotline, 140
neighborhood watch, 155
neighbors, and self-care, 99
noises, normal, 97
"No one will believe you," 60

obedience, blind:
   vs. respect, 44
   vs. safety, 123–25
offenders:
   "badness" and, 48
   boyfriends as, 43–44
   children as, 44–45
   defined, 65
   and emotional coercion, 60
   grooming process of, 45
   in incest, 43
   intimidation by, 123
   pedophiles, 42, 66
   responsibility of, 143
   in sexual abuse, 42–43
   stepparents as, 43–44
   and stereotypes, 68
   and strangers, see strangers
   telephone calls from, 94–95
   testing by, 45
   threats from, 60
   tools of, 45, 60, 66
   treatment programs for, 142

and unoccupied homes, 95–96
visual clues to, 67–68, 145

parents:
   ambivalence of, 7–8
   of bullying child, 103–6
   child's expectations for, 83
   expectations of, 90
   and Internet, see Internet
   listening and, 63–64
   partnership with, 86
   as protectors, 146
   and reporting abuse, 140–42
   response of, 138–39
   rural, 89
   school communication with, 153
   as school volunteers, 156, 160
   suburban, 89
   support and help from, 142–43,
      155
   urban, 89
   in "What If . . ." game, 34–37
   see also adults
Parents on Patrol (POP), 155
pass system, in school, 157
pedophiles, 42, 66
peer pressure, 32, 56–57
perpetrators, see offenders
pickups, during and after school,
   157–58
playground aides, 108, 156
playground equipment, 156
playground security, 152–54, 156
playing sex vs. playing doctor, 47,
   48–49
politeness vs. safety, 77, 121–22
POP (Parents on Patrol), 155
pornography, on Internet, 115–16
power, physical, 32
prank telephone calls, 94
preschoolers:
   Arm's Reach Plus rule for, 73–
      75
   as most teachable moment, 14
   and prevention, 56
   "What If . . ." game for, 31

preteens:
  Arm's Reach Plus rule for, 76
  and communication, 32–33
  embarrassment of, 32, 56–57, 76
  independence sought by, 32
  and peer pressure, 32, 56–57
  and prevention, 56–58
  "What If . . ." game for, 32–33
prevention, 20–24, 50–64, 72–87
  and adult response, 55–58
  Arm's Reach Plus rule, 72–76
  attracting attention, 85
  and body language, 52
  and body parts, 52–53
  of bullying, 104–8
  code word and, 84, 117, 158
  and communication, 58, 63–64
  defined, 40
  Don't Go Anywhere with a
    Stranger rule, 82–83
  Don't Take Things from Strangers
    rule, 79–82
  Don't Talk to Strangers rule, 77–79
  and double messages, 53–55
  effectiveness of, 13–16
  of emotional coercion, 60
  experience as base for, 14
  and fear tactics, 67
  and Internet, see Internet
  and mixed messages, 53–55
  most teachable moment for, 14
  one-shot efforts toward, 13–14
  ownership of body and, 50–51
  and politeness, 77, 121–22
  practicing skills of, 58
  principles of, 51
  and rules for adults, 62–63,
    145–50
  safety without fear, 17–19
  and saying no, see saying no
  scare tactics in, 18
  in schools, see schools
  and secrets, 61–62
  and seven- to sixteen-year-olds,
    56–58
  and tattling, 59

  and telling, 58–59, 63–64
  and three- to six-year-olds, 56
  touching and, 50–51, 55
  and whom to tell, 63–64
  see also "What If . . ." game
privacy vs. secrecy, 62
private parts, 52–53
promises, breaking, 122–23
protectors, parents as, 146
provocative behavior, 47, 102

questions:
  inappropriate, 34, 35–36
  repetitious, 33–34
  "silly," 34
  in telephone calls, 95
  underlying concerns in, 34

reality vs. make-believe, 32, 46–47
relationship, in sexual abuse, 46
reports of child abuse, 139–41
  false, 46–47
  hotline for, 140
  and interviews of child, 141
  mandatory, 141, 152
  in media, 47
  parental control of, 140–42
  and therapy, 142–44
resources:
  for help, 99
  Internet, 116
respect vs. blind obedience, 44
responsibility:
  of adults, 145–50
  of children, 18, 69–70, 86
  of offenders, 143
  privileges and, 92
  see also self-care
robberies, and self-care, 97–98
role-play:
  and Arm's Reach Plus rule, 74
  and bullies, 104
  and Don't Take Things from
    Strangers rule, 80, 81
  in prevention education, 14
  and "What If . . ." game, 29

rudeness vs. safety, 77, 121–22
rules:
  for adults, 62–63, 145–50
  Arm's Reach Plus, 72–76
  and blind obedience, 123–25
  and breaking promises, 122–23
  checklist of, 87
  difficulty of following, 80–81
  Don't Go Anywhere with a
    Stranger, 82–83
  Don't Take Things from
    Strangers, 79–82
  Don't Talk to Strangers, 77–79
  in emergencies, 98
  exceptions to, 120–25
  for Internet use, 116–17
  and lying, 122–23
  and politeness, 121–22
  and saying no, 125
  for self-care, 90–92
  and strangers, 72–83, 87
  and trust, 125
runaways, 64

Safe Child Program, 15–16, 161–62
safety:
  vs. blind obedience, 123–25
  circle of, 72
  on Internet, 115–16, 118
  lying and, 122–23
  vs. politeness, 77, 121–22
  in schools, *see* schools
  without fear, 17–19
sales offers, on Internet, 117
sales telephone calls, 94–95
saying no:
  and being hurt, 59
  permission for, 34–35, 52, 58,
    148
  and rules, 125
  to touching, 50–51, 52, 56, 58
scare tactics:
  ineffectiveness of, 18
  vs. Safe Child approach, 67
  and "What if . . ." game, 28–30
  see also fear

schools, 151–62
  absence from, 158
  after-school programs, 152–53
  and bullying, 108
  bus to, 154–55
  call system in, 158
  on campus, 157
  and code word, 84, 158
  communication with parents
    from, 153
  employees of, 151–52
  field trips of, 79, 159
  identification of guests in, 157
  locked buildings of, 157
  mandatory reporting law and,
    152
  neighborhood watch and, 155
  Parents on Patrol and, 155
  pass system in, 157
  pickups during and after, 157–58
  playground aides, 108, 156
  playground equipment of, 156
  playground security of, 152–54,
    156
  prevention programs in, 159
  substitutes in, 158
  supervision in, 152, 156
  walking to, 154–55
  working together with, 160
secrets:
  children and, 61–62
  and "I'm going to tell," 62
  vs. privacy, 62
  vs. surprises, 61
  touching and, 62
security:
  on playgrounds, 152–54, 156
  in schools, 157
self-care, 69–70, 88–99
  answering machines, 93
  answering the door, 95–96
  answering the telephone, 92–95
  checklist, 91
  and emergencies, 97–98
  expectations vs. performance in,
    90

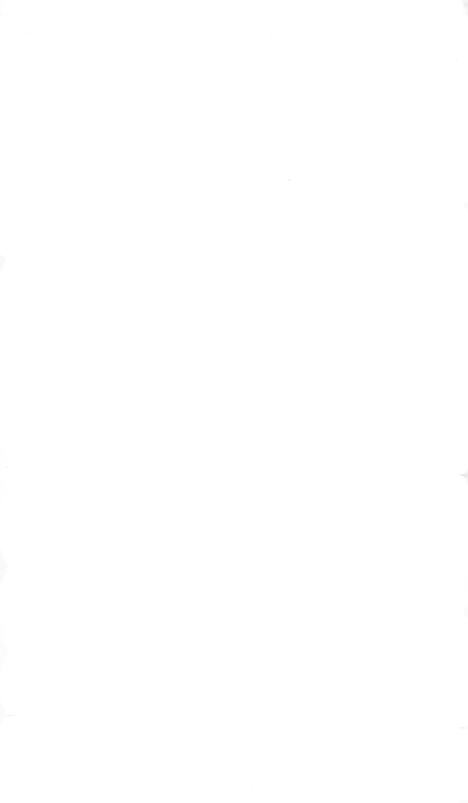

8883235R0

Made in the USA
Lexington, KY
10 March 2011